# PHYSICAL THERAPY
# PROCEDURES

*Third Edition, Second Printing*

# PHYSICAL THERAPY PROCEDURES

## Selected Techniques

*By*

**ANN H. DOWNER, B.A., M.S., L.P.T.**

*Associate Professor*
*College of Medicine*
*School of Allied Medical Professions*
*Physical Therapy Division*
*The Ohio State University*
*Columbus, Ohio*

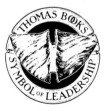

**CHARLES C THOMAS • PUBLISHER**
*Springfield • Illinois • U.S.A.*

*Published and Distributed Throughout the World by*

CHARLES  C  THOMAS  •  PUBLISHER

Bannerstone House

301-327 East Lawrence Avenue, Springfield, Illinois, U.S.A.

First Edition, First Printing, 1970
First Edition, Second Printing, 1971
First Edition, Third Printing, 1973
Second Edition, First Printing, 1974
Second Edition, Second Printing, 1975
Second Edition, Third Printing, 1977
Third Edition, First Printing, 1978
Third Edition, Second Printing, 1981

*Printed in the United States of America*
*V-R-1*

*Library of Congress Cataloging in Publication Data*

Downer, Ann H
   Physical therapy procedures.

Bibliography: p. 295
   Includes index.
   1. Physical therapy.  I. Title.  [DNLM:  1. Phys-
ical therapy.  WB460 D748p]
RM700.D73 1979        615'.8        78-15492
ISBN 0-398-03840-6

# PREFACE TO THE THIRD EDITION

THERE are many arguments against the writing and printing of a new edition of any book. One of these is the cost in time and money. It costs far less to reprint an old edition than it does to print a completely revised edition, and the time it takes to improve and update a manuscript is almost as much as it took to write the book in the first place.

There were several deciding factors for a new edition. One was the necessity of including a new technique, Myofeedback, and adding an old technique, Transcutaneous Electrical Nerve Stimulation. TENS (TNS) is by no means new as both direct current by itself and with modulations as well as low frequency alternating current have been used to treat pain and other patient problems in the physical therapy department for many years. However, the advent of the mini electrical stimulation units that enable the patients to treat themselves at home has provided the use of electricity with a new popularity, and TENS has gained a new prominence in the treatment repertoire of the physical therapist.

As the book has been used over the years, students and therapists have offered valuable suggestions and constructive criticisms. These combined with the author's own experience have made it necessary to rewrite almost every chapter. New illustrations have been added, which should facilitate use of the book.

This kind of book does not rival some of the textbooks listed in the bibliography. It is still a "how to" book, a step-by-step procedure for applying modalities and nothing more. Even though the "how to" of operating any unit is a very small part of the total knowledge necessary to treat patients, it represents a very large part of the patient's safety. The total practice of physical therapy is a blending of many facets. This is only one.

The author gratefully acknowledges the physical therapists,

students, and athletic trainers who offered suggestions; Gary Bowman, Maryclare Burgett, Robert Mace, Leesa Nystrom, Gretchen Owen, Susan Rousch, and Susan Willett — physical therapy students; Miss Mary Ellen Keil who posed for pictures; and the many manufacturers who generously allowed use of their equipment photographs.

A.H.D.

# PREFACE TO THE SECOND EDITION

"A COOKBOOK on Physical Therapy" was a phrase used to describe the first edition, and the author considers this to be an excellent description. As was the first edition, the second edition, which is appearing approximately three years after the first edition, is a "how to" book and nothing more. The student must learn to think for himself, evaluate the effectiveness of treatment and analyze procedures, but these abilities come with a total learning process and experience. This book presents only a very small part of the knowledge the student must acquire in the use of modalities.

Because of the many valuable suggestions from students and therapists, the first edition has been extensively revised and two new chapters have been added. Set-up pictures have been included which will provide visibility to certain techniques.

The author wishes to extend her sincere thanks for the many helpful comments and constructive criticisms which have been used in revising the book.

A special thank-you goes to Miss Gladys G. Woods, Director, Division of Physical Therapy, The Ohio State University, for her continued encouragement and help. I am indebted to Mrs. Marilyn Fetters, a graduate student, Physical Therapy Division, The Ohio State University, for the many hours she spent posing for the set-up pictures. My secretary, Mrs. Dora Curtin, has done an excellent job of typing the manuscript.

Again, Mr. Payne Thomas of Charles C Thomas, Publisher has been very patient in answering my many questions.

A.H.D.

# PREFACE TO THE FIRST EDITION

THIS manual brings together in one book most of the common techniques used in various modalities. Many of the procedures have been used to treat patients for many years, and it is expected they will be used for many years to come. Some new modalities are included which require basically the same techniques while other modalities require new techniques.

The author does not wish to suggest that one technique may be better than another or that one particular piece of equipment will give more beneficial results than another. No attempt has been made to discuss the physics, effects, indications, or contraindications. Rather, the manual outlines in detail a step-by-step procedure which may be followed with each technique to ensure the patient's safety and comfort and, hopefully, to relieve his symptoms.

The manual should prove particularly useful to the students in the field of physical therapy and their instructors, to physicians and nurses, and to athletic trainers and their athletes.

The author wishes to express her sincere appreciation to those who have read the manuscript and given suggestions: Gladys G. Woods, Director, Division of Physical Therapy, The Ohio State University; Marian Chase, Chief Physical Therapist, Mental Retardation Program, The Ohio State University; and Rebecca Fauser, Mickey Galleher, Fred Hershberger, Mary Hopper, and Paul Mitchell, physical therapy students at The Ohio State University.

Mr. Payne Thomas of Charles C Thomas, Publisher has given me valuable advice and assistance.

I am indebted to the many manufacturers who have given their permission to use printed material and pictures.

A.H.D.

# CONTENTS

## Part IV
## Cold Techniques

## Part V
## Electricity Techniques

## Part VI
## Ultraviolet Techniques

## Part VII
## Traction Techniques

# Part VIII
## Miscellaneous Techniques

# PHYSICAL THERAPY
# PROCEDURES

# Part I
## Introduction

## Chapter 1

# GENERAL CONSIDERATIONS FOR ALL TREATMENTS

## *I. Preparations*

A.  The therapist:
1.  Your clothing should be neat and clean and should allow freedom of movement:
    a.  Washable, permanent press material is the most economical.
    b.  Sleeves should be loose and no longer than three-quarter length.
    c.  Shoes should be comfortable and have resilient and skid resistent soles and heels.
2.  Your hair should be clean and short or tied back so it will not interfere with the treatment or touch the patient or the unit.
3.  Use a deodorant and guard against bad breath.
4.  Do not wear jewelry other than a watch and wedding ring:
    a.  Jewelry can be extremely dangerous around electrical equipment.
    b.  An inexpensive, nonmagnetic, water resistant watch with a sweep second hand is recommended. A stretch band will allow for pushing the watch up your arm rather than removing it for some treatments.
    c.  A digital watch is not recommended unless seconds can be read without having to hold in a button.
    d.  An expensive watch can easily be ruined by accidental immersion in water, by being magnetized, etc.
5.  Do not use strongly scented creams, lotions, hair sprays, after shave lotions, etc.
6.  Your hands should be washed before each patient is treated, and your nails should be short and clean.

       7. Malpractice insurance is an excellent investment.

B.   Nonverbal communications:

    1. In addition to cleanliness and neatness, other types of nonverbal communication can establish a supportive setting for treatment:

       a. Touch. Greet the patient with a handshake. Touching an amputation stump or a paralyzed leg indicates acceptance. However, avoid touching the genital/breast area unless indicated for treatment. Help the patient only when necessary.

       b. Lowering yourself. To lessen the superior-subordinate relationship, stoop or bend to greet a patient if he is in a wheelchair, on a cart, or shorter than you. Squat to greet a child if he is walking. Hold an infant in your lap and play with him before attempting to treat him. When possible, sit to treat any patient.

       c. Smile with your eyes as well as with your mouth.

       d. Look the patient directly in the eye when you talk. Do *not* look at the eyelid, forehead, or off into space.

       e. Talk *with* the patient, not to him.

       f. Focus your attention on *that* patient.

C.   Patient-therapist rapport:

    1. By the very nature of the situation, you are in a position of authority. Use it wisely.

    2. *Every* patient is an individual. Treat him as such.

    3. Be understanding, but not personal.

    4. Avoid controversial subjects unless you agree with the patient.

    5. *Never* discuss your personal problems with the patient. He is interested in his problems, not yours.

    6. Discuss his condition only as it relates to his treatment and progress. It is *not* your prerogative to tell a patient he will not walk again, he has a certain disease, he is dying, etc.

    7. Do *not* criticize the patient's physician or other personnel.

    8. If the patient is not happy with his physician, suggest

that he discuss with his physician the wish for another opinion on his problem.

9. Tell the truth. If a treatment may cause pain, do *not* tell the patient it will not hurt.
10. Confidences are sacred. If you feel the patient's physician should know what the patient has told you, persuade the patient to tell his doctor himself.
11. Do *not* accept gifts or money from patients.
12. Respect age.
13. Really *care* about each patient.
14. Always treat the patient in the physical therapy department when using modality equipment.

D. Review the patient's medical record:
   1. History, physical findings, drugs, admission data, etc.
   2. Diagnosis:
      a. If possible, you should know what the diagnosis is *before* you treat the patient. Some diagnoses will preclude the use of certain modalities, types of treatment, etc.
      b. The physician should notify you if there is any change in the diagnosis.
      c. It is your responsibility to provide the patient's physician with any information that may assist in making (changing) the diagnosis.
   3. Prescription for treatment:
      a. It is not only your prerogative, but your responsibility to question any prescription for treatment.
      b. If the qualified physical therapist prescribes the treatment, he must be aware of the implications of using the wrong modality.
   4. Contraindications:
      a. You must know whether or not any contraindications preclude the use of a specific modality.
      b. It is your responsibility to advise the physician when the requested treatment is contraindicated or inadvisable.
      c. It is your responsibility to refuse to carry out a prescribed treatment if you feel it is contraindicated or

inadvisable.
5. Special problems:
   a. Handling and/or treatment of patients with special problems such as deafness or blindness may have to be modified.
   b. Be *sure* to check the patient and/or his medical record for any external or implanted electrical or atomic stimulation devices such as transcutaneous nerve stimulators, lung or bladder stimulators, heart pacemakers, and any implanted metal, as these are contraindications for some modalities.
E. Determine the procedure to be used:
  1. Type of modality, technique, equipment needed.
  2. Patient's position for treatment.
  3. Draping procedure.
  4. Position of the unit in relation to the patient.
  5. Treatment time.
  6. Etc.
F. Prepare the treatment area:
  1. The treatment area should be enclosed to guarantee privacy for the patient. Curtains should be equipped with a snap clothespin or a snap to prevent gapping during treatment.
  2. Unless the patient is to be treated on a cart, a plinth should be in the cubicle:
   a. The plinth should be made entirely of wood.
   b. Plinth measurements should be 30 inches wide by 72 to 76 inches long by 30 to 32 inches high. To increase the height of the plinth, boxes may be built for each, leg.
   c. The plinth pad or mattress and covering should be clean, and they should not contain any metal.
   d. If possible, the plinth should be placed on the side of the booth opposite the opening in the curtains.
   e. Place the plinth close to the wall and curtains to allow as much space as possible for the patient and the unit.
   f. Make sure the plinth does not extend into the aisle

or another treatment cubicle. The plinth must also be placed so the patient's feet (head) will not be in the aisle or in another treatment cubicle.

3. A wood chair should be in the cubicle (unless the patient is to be treated on a cart or while seated in his wheelchair):
   a. The chair is for the patient, and it should not be used for linen, pillows or equipment.
   b. Put the chair in a convenient place, but keep it away from the unit to be used.
   c. If the patient is to sit in the chair for his treatment, place the chair in its final position.
4. There should be no modality equipment in the cubicle other than the equipment you will use:
   a. Put the unit at the back of the cubicle out of the patient's way.
   b. Direct lamps away from the treatment area.
   c. Preheat the unit if indicated.
5. A footstool should be readily available.
6. Check the floor to be sure it is completely dry.
7. Collect all linens, pillows, and equipment:
   a. Keep all extra linens, pillows and equipment on the plinth shelf and not on the chair, plinth, or unit.
   b. A minimum of two pillows is essential.

G. Prepare the plinth:
1. All linen should be clean for each patient.
2. If the patient is to be in the prone position, pull down the plinth pad just enough to pad the end of the plinth.
3. Place support pillows in the correct positions (see II. L, M, and N.)
4. Unfold the drape sheet and spread it lengthwise on the far side of the plinth *over* the knee/abdomen pillow.

H. Electrical safety:
1. Know where the fire extinguishers are for each kind of fire and know how to use them.
2. Use only equipment with three wire line cords. If using old equipment, be sure it is properly grounded. Converter plugs may be used, but only as a temporary mea-

sure.

3. A short line cord is preferable to a long one because current leakage is less.
4. *Never* use extension cords.
5. *Never* use a metal plinth, chair, or table or one with metal legs or arms.
6. *Never* treat a patient who is lying on an innerspring mattress with short wave diathermy or microwave.
7. Kinked wires or line cords are suspect. Do *not* use them.
8. Do *not* touch electrodes on any unit while manipulating the controls on an operating unit.
9. An unusual noise such as a buzzing sound, unusual odors, tingling sensations where there are not supposed to be any, frayed line cords, etc. are contraindications for using that unit.
10. Do not touch any metal such as water faucets, sinks, radiators, or beds while using electrical units, and do not let operating units touch any metal.
11. Do *not* remove line cords from a wall/floor receptacle by holding onto the wire.
12. Touch only one piece of operating equipment at any one time.
13. Do not plug in or unplug one unit while touching another operating unit.
14. *Never* attempt to repair equipment unless you are trained to do so.
15. *Never* use two electrical modality units on one patient at the same time.
16. *Electricity can kill you and the patient. Do not take chances.*

I.  Check the unit:
    1. Know how to operate the unit. *Never* use a modality unit on a patient until you are *thoroughly* familiar with its operation.
    2. *Never* use defective equipment (see Electrical safety):
       a. All electrical connections should be tight.
       b. All manual and automatic adjustments must be in proper working order.

3. All necessary parts should be ready to use.
4. Warm up the unit if necessary.
5. When adjusting electrodes, raising lamps, etc., always loosen the adjustment knobs.
6. Test the unit on yourself to be sure it is operating safely and efficiently.

## II. Starting the Treatment

A. Know *exactly* what you are going to do and how to do it:
   1. If in doubt, find out *before* the patient comes in for treatment.
   2. *Never* use any modality unit until you know *exactly* how to operate it and you are aware of all of the ramifications of using that particular unit.
B. You may require assistance with some patients or modalities. Have another staff member (not a patient or a patient's relative) ready to assist you when in doubt:
   1. *Never* attempt to lift a patient unless it is absolutely necessary.
   2. If using a large unit such as a body baker, always have a staff member help you to lessen the chance of dropping the unit on the patient.
C. Be calm and reassuring while setting up and administering the treatment:
   1. Many patients, especially children, may be extremely apprehensive about being hurt, being treated with impressive equipment, meeting new people, etc. Your composure and quiet efficiency will help allay any fears and apprehension.
   2. Motivating the patient and gaining his confidence will aid the effectiveness of the treatment.
D. Give the patient your name and be sure he knows it:
   1. When pain or discomfort occurs, some patients will be reluctant to call you if they do not know your name. Emphasize that he should call out to anyone if he does not remember your name.
   2. You should know the patient's name and know how to pronounce it correctly.

3. Miss, Mr. or Mrs. is preferable when addressing adults.
4. Children should address you as "Miss Mary" or "Mr. Ryan," as parents may be trying to train them.

E. Begin to evaluate the patient as he comes in for treatment:
   1. Female or male.
   2. Young, old, middle age.
   3. Tall, short, fat, thin.
   4. Two eyes, two ears, two noses.
   5. Hair, color, long, short, wig.
   6. Hospital gown, street clothes.
   7. Smiling, crying, in pain, defensive, afraid.
   8. Walking unaided, crutches, cane, normal gait, limp, etc.
   9. In wheelchair, on cart.
  10. General skin color, tan, blotchy, red, etc.
  11. Casts, slings, braces.
  12. Posture, deformity, body asymmetry.
  13. Can patient see, hear, communicate, understand, etc.
  14. Psychotic, retarded, senile, just plain odd.
  15. Etc.

F. Direct the patient into a treatment cubicle.

G. Explain the procedure to the patient:
   1. Tell him what you are going to do. Use correct, simple and positive terms.
   2. Describe the sensation he *should* feel:
     a. Do not scare the patient.
     b. Do *not* lie to the patient.
   3. Tell him how long the treatment will be.
   4. Impress him with the importance of calling you/ someone *immediately* if *any* discomfort occurs:
     a. Any burning sensation from a heat or electrical treatment.
     b. Pain, dizziness, faintness, or any other untoward symptoms.
     c. If he has to move from the position in which you placed him, he should call you *before* he moves:
       1. Explain why he should call you before he moves:
       2. This will not occur if you have initially provided

    adequate pillow support with proper positioning.

   d. He should call you if he is cold.

  5. Tell the patient what the skin will look like after treatment.

H. Instruct (help) the patient to remove his clothing:

  1. Give clear, slow, and sufficient instructions.

  2. Do *not* help the patient unless his disability, general condition, or age warrant′ aid.

  3. The patient *must* remove all clothing from the part to be treated. If he will not remove his clothing, do *not* treat him.

  4. For treatments to patients who will by lying on the plinth, *all outer* clothing (trousers, dresses, skirts, blouses, shirts, etc.) should be removed to prevent them from becoming soiled from lotions, gels, etc., wrinkled, or wet from water or perspiration.

  5. Shoes should be removed if the patient is on the plinth whether or not the feet are going to be treated.

  6. Remove any constricting clothing.

  7. *Never* allow a patient to roll up a sleeve or pant leg as this can impair circulation.

  8. For general heat treatments, have the patient completely undress, and provide him with appropriate substitutes such as a gown, T-binder, etc.

  9. Provide hangers, hooks, etc. so the patient may hang his clothes.

  10. Report to your supervisor any patient who unnecessarily exposes himself/herself.

I. All braces, splints, bandages, etc. should be removed if appropriate and if not contraindicated.

J. Valuables:

  1. Have the patient remove his jewelry *before* he gets into the treatment position.

  2. Rings, watches, necklaces, ear studs, etc. must *always* be removed from the area being treated and in appropriate instances:

   a. Watches can be magnetized by short wave diathermy and microwave. They can get wet, etc.

   b. Any metal is a real danger in the vicinity of elec-
      tricity.
   3. Keep the patient's valuables with him:
      a. Have him put them in a pocket or purse; if you do
         it, have him watch you.
      b. Do *not* put his valuables in your pocket.
      c. If the patient forgets any valuables, take them to
         him if he is an inpatient. If he is an outpatient, put
         them in the hospital/clinic safe and get a receipt. Do
         *not* keep them in your desk drawer even though you
         can lock it.
K. Place the patient in the postion that will be comfortable
   throughout the treatment and that will enable you to treat
   the part safely and efficiently:
   1. The patient's prescription, disability, general condi-
      tion, and age will determine his position.
   2. His position should allow effective and safe use of the
      equipment. The length of the line cord is an important
      consideration when positioning the patient.
   3. His position should provide for your good body me-
      chanics:
      a. Put him close to the side of the plinth from which
         you will do the massage/exercise, etc.
      b. You should sit to treat the patient whenever pos-
         sible.
   4. The patient must be as relaxed as possible.
   5. Do *not* place the patient in such a position that a part
      of him will protrude into another treatment cubicle or
      the aisle.
L. The sitting position:
   1. The patient should lie down when the chest, pelvis,
      low back, or lower extremities are to be treated.
   2. If possible, never treat a patient while he is sitting on
      the end or side of the plinth, long sitting on the plinth,
      or sitting on the plinth with a wall supporting his
      back. If the plinth is hinged in the middle so one half
      of it can be used as a back rest, the patient may then sit
      on the plinth with a pillow under his knees.

3. Use a chair with a back rest:
   a. The chair should be low/high enough to allow the patient's feet to rest comfortably on the floor.
   b. If the chair is too high, give the patient a footstool.
4. The patient may sit facing the plinth:
   a. His knees should be able to go under the plinth.

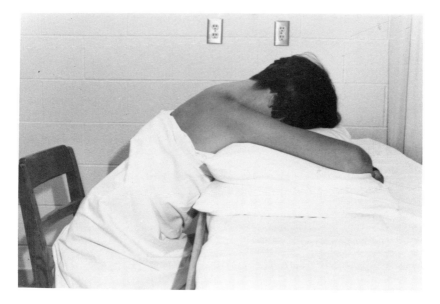

Figure 1. Facing the plinth.

   b. His elbows and forearms should rest comfortably on the plinth. The chair must be high enough. If not, let him sit on a pillow.
   c. If treating the neck and/or upper back, provide pillows on which the patient may rest his head. If muscle spasm or tight muscles are present, more than one pillow may be necessary.
5. The patient may sit with his side next to the end or side of the plinth:
   a. He should sit with his involved upper extremity next to the plinth.
   b. Support the involved extremity on the plinth. The

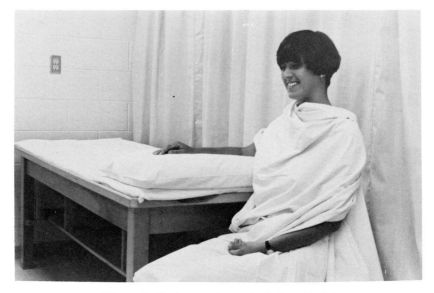

Figure 2. Sitting at the end of the plinth.

chair must be high enough, or have the patient sit on a pillow.

  c. A pillow in the patient's lap to support the uninvolved extremity may help relax the patient.

  d. If stretching of the involved extremity is desired, put a pillow under that extremity on the plinth.

  e. A pillow should be used to support the forearm when the shoulder is externally rotated and the forearm is in supination.

  f. The hand should be supported with a rolled towel when the forearm is supinated and resting on the plinth.

M. The supine position:

  1. The patient's head can be put at either end of the plinth.

  2. The patient's involved side should be closest to the therapist.

  3. The patient should be close to the edge of the plinth to allow you to use good body mechanics.

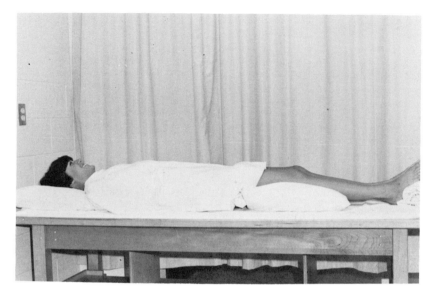

Figure 3. The supine position.

4. One pillow should be under the patient's head:
   a. More than one pillow may be needed.
   b. Placing a pillow under the head and shoulders may be more comfortable for selected patients.
5. One or two pillows should be under the patient's knees:
   a. Flexion of the hips is essential to reduce the lumbar curve.
   b. The use of pillows may be contraindicated as with hip/knee flexion contractures.
6. If decubitae are present on the heels, rolled towels under the ankles will relieve pressure. Care must be taken not to put the knees into hyperextension.

N. The prone position:
1. The patient's head may be put at either end of the plinth:
   a. No pillow should be used under the head or chest.
2. A large pillow should go under the patient's abdomen to reduce the lumbar curve:
   a. Some patients may require two pillows.

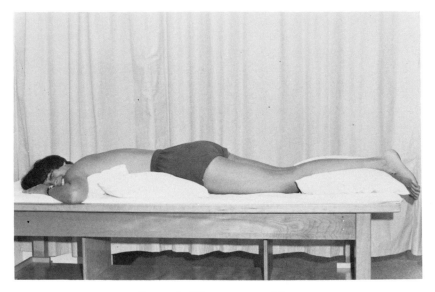

Figure 4. The prone position.

    b. Flexion and external rotation of the hip and flexion of the knee on the same side to which the patient's head is turned may be more comfortable than completely extended lower extremities.

3. The patient's involved side should be nearest the therapist.
4. The patient should be close to the edge of the plinth to allow you to use good body mechanics.
5. The patient's feet and ankles should go off the end of the plinth to the level of the malleoli to prevent plantar flexion. The plinth pad should be pulled down to pad the foot edge of the plinth.
6. When treating the hamstring and/or calf areas, a pillow under the leg (do not include the knee or foot) or rolled towels under the ankles will provide relaxation by flexing the knees.
7. A pillow under the tip of the shoulder on the side to which the patient's head is turned may help breathing.
8. Rolled towels at the side of the trunk in the axillae will

shield the breast area of women.

O. The sidelying position:
1. The patient's head may go at either end of the plinth.
2. Place a thick pillow or a thin pillow folded in half under the patient's head to "fill up" the space between the head and shoulder.

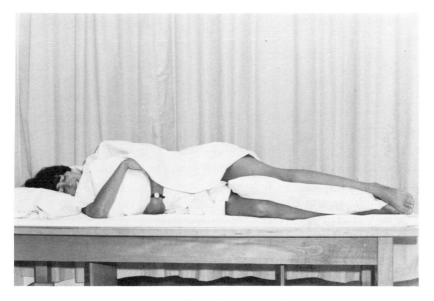

Figure 5. The sidelying position.

3. The hips and knees should be flexed from 70 to 90 degrees to provide a wide base of support.
4. Place a large pillow lengthwise between the knees and the medial malleoli to relieve pressure and to reduce adduction of the uppermost hip:
   a. If treating the uppermost hip or if the bottom hip is flexed or extended more than the upper hip, use two pillows under the uppermost thigh.
5. Give the patient a large pillow to "hug."
P. Draping:
1. Respect the patient's modesty. When clothes must be removed, the patient should be treated in private and he

should *always* be properly draped. Other patients, staff members, or visitors may inadvertently look into the treatment cubicle. A patient should never be treated in the nude unless it is absolutely necessary.

2. The amount and method of draping depend on:
   a. The position of the patient.
   b. The area being treated.
   c. The amount of clothing that must be removed.
   d. The temperature of the room.
   e. The age of the patient.
3. Provide the patient with a large drape sheet or cotton bath blanket. It should be completely unfolded and put lengthwise over any support pillows.
4. *Tell* the patient to cover himself with the drape sheet after he has removed his clothing.
5. The draping should be secure but not tight.
6. The patient should not have to hold the draping around him. Tucking in or taping are the best ways to secure the draping. (Pins or any metal are contraindicated with certain treatments.)
7. Use heavy turkish toweling or terry cloth to cover genital and/or breast areas. These areas should *never* be exposed unless it is necessary for treatment.
8. If you have to rearrange the draping, keep your hands away from the genital and breast areas.
9. Make sure the patient is warm throughout the treatment:
   a. Use extra sheets and towels if necessary.
   b. Do *not* use infrared lamps or any other heat modality to keep the patient warm.

Q. Ask the patient to tell you where he has pain:
   1. The area where there is pain does not necessarily mean that this will be the area to be treated, and an explanation to the patient may be necessary.
R. Patient examination:
   1. Be *sure* you treat the correct area:
      a. If the prescription calls for the cervical area to be

treated, do not treat the upper back; if the left ankle is to be treated, do not treat the right ankle, etc.

   b. Some electrodes/packs, etc. may be too large to treat one specific area.

2. Expose only the area to be treated.

3. Check the skin on the area to be treated:
   a. Skin color — pale, flushed, blue, mottled, etc.
   b. Skin rash.
   c. Skin integrity.
   d. Recent scars, new skin.
   e. Moles, etc.

4. Check skin sensation:
   a. Ask the patient to close his eyes. Run your finger over the skin and ask the patient if he can feel it.
   b. The diagnosis may indicate sensory changes.
   c. Almost any modality must be used with *extreme* caution or not at all when sensation is lacking or diminished.
   d. Ask the patient if he has any problem distinguishing heat and cold.

5. Note any bone or joint deviations.

6. Note any edema. Soft tissue edema and/or tenderness may be contraindications for some modalities.

7. Check joint range of motion in the area to be treated as well as immediately above and below.

8. Is there pain on movement? Some patients are embarrassed to admit they have pain. Watch their eyes, as they are good indicators of pain.

9. A gross evaluation of muscle strength is helpful.

10. Note any muscle atrophy, hypertrophy, etc.

11. Note breathing ability.

12. Be *sure* to check the patient and/or his medical records for any external or implanted electrical stimulation devices such as transcutaneous nerve stimulators, lung or bladder stimulators, heart pacemakers, hearing aides, etc. as these are contraindications for some modalities.

S. If you have any doubts about treating the patient, check

with your supervisor.

T. Establish realistic treatment goals for the patient, both short term and long term. Goals provide incentives for the patient. They must be attainable and they must be established in relation to:
    1. The patient's diagnosis.
    2. The patient's general condition.
    3. The patient's age.
    4. The specific disability.
    5. Available equipment.
    6. The specific modality to be used for treatment.
    7. Time available for treatment.
    8. Dangers.
    9. Contraindications.
    10. The patient's expectations for himself.

U. Position the unit (electrodes, packs, etc.) and turn on the unit, unless preheated.

V. Set an interval timer or take note of the time. The treatment time will vary according to the modality used and the condition of the patient.

W. Once again, instruct the patient to call you if he has pain, is uncomfortable for any reason, etc. Remind him to call out to anyone if he cannot remember your name. Reassure him that someone will be within hearing distance throughout his entire treatment.

X. Tell him you will check back with him occasionally to be sure all is well.

Y. If the patient becomes faint, nauseated, overheated, etc., or in case of an emergency, terminate treatment.

### III. Terminating the Treatment

A. Turn off the unit, remove the electrodes, etc., and move the unit to the back of the cubicle out of the patient's way. Put packs on the plinth shelf, etc. Take care of the patient before cleaning up the equipment and the cubicle.

B. Give the patient a clean, dry turkish towel and have (help) him thoroughly dry his skin:

1. If he cannot reach the area, has too much pain, etc., dry his skin for him.
2. To remove oil, pour some alcohol onto the towel (not onto the patient) and let the patient clean his skin.

C. Re-evaluate the patient:
   1. Check the skin for any unusual marks that were not there before treatment. If you find any, tell your supervisor, the patient's physician, or any physician *immediately*. Do *not* allow the patient to leave the department until action has been taken.
   2. If the patient has become overheated for any reason, if he does not feel well, has pain, etc., have him sit on the edge of the plinth for a few seconds to be sure he is not dizzy or does not feel faint:
      a. Be sure he remains properly draped.
      b. Stand directly in front of him to prevent him from falling forward. Remember that he could also fall backward.
      c. Do not allow him to become chilled.

D. If no further treatment is to follow, give him his clothes and tell him to dress.
E. If an outpatient is very warm, urge him to sit in the waiting room for five to ten minutes to cool off before going outside.
F. Tell the patient the day and hour to return or have him check with the receptionist.
G. Remove the unit, pack, etc., and prepare the area for the next treatment.
H. Record the treatment and progress notes on the patient's hospital and/or physical therapy department records.

## *IV. Number of Treatments*

A. The number of treatments per day/week as well as the total number of treatments should be included on the prescription for treatment:
   1. The number of treatments per day/week will vary with the individual physician, the patient's condition, avail-

able time, number of therapists, etc.
2. The patient should be checked by his physician:
   a. At least every two weeks if the problem is acute, and every month in chronic problems.
   b. Whenever untoward symptoms occur, such as an increase in pain, adverse reaction to treatment, etc.

## *IV. Home Treatments*

A. Written instructions for the patient are essential. These may be printed instructions, or sometimes it is more meaningful if the patient writes the instructions.
B. The instructions should include:
   1. Why the patient should continue the treatment at home.
   2. Exact and sequential directions for using each particular motality.
   3. How long each treatment should be.
   4. The patient's exact position explaining the use of pillows, firm surface, body position, etc.
   5. Exact sensations the patient should feel.
   6. What he should not feel.
   7. Precautions, dangers, contraindications.
   8. How many times per day the treatment should be done.
   9. How many times per week the treatment should be done.
   10. The date the patient should return for a recheck by the physical therapist/physician.
C. Tell the patient that no other member of his family should use any modality unit.
D. Tell him to contact you if any untoward symptoms develop.
E. The patient should always practice the procedure in the department before he goes home.

## *V. Precautions*

A. Be alert and prevent accidents.

B. When burns or other problems occur, report them to your supervisor or to the patient's physician (or to any physician in an emergency) *immediately;*
   1. Know how to call a physician to your department. Do *not* wait until an emergency occurs to learn how to do this.
C. The patient should *not* leave the department until the accident has been reported and action instituted.
D. Record the following on the patient's hospital and/or physical therapy records:
   1. What the problem is.
   2. *Exactly* where the burn occurred. Be *extremely* specific, such as "the anterior surface, distal end of the right thigh 3 inches above the patella."
   3. What modality was used.
   4. The distance, intensity, etc. as applicable.
   5. What instructions had been given to the patient before treatment.
   6. Whether or not you had checked the patient periodically throughout the treatment.
   7. The exact time the accident occurred.
   8. The correct date.
   9. What was done, such as a physician was called, bandage was applied, etc.
   10. Your signature.
   11. Physician's signature.
   12. Any witnesses names should be recorded.
E. It may be necessary, and usually is, to fill out an accident report:
   1. Follow hospital and/or department regulations.
   2. Fill out the report as soon as the patient leaves the department while the events, time, etc. are fresh in your mind. The report could be used in any ensuing litigation.
   3. Accuracy and attention to detail are essential.
F. Treatment with *any* modality should *always* be safe and comfortable for the patient.
G. Terminate treatment any time dizziness, nausea, faintness,

tiredness, pain, overheating, or other untoward symptoms develop.

H.  Treatment may have to be modified for the very young, very old, psychotic, retarded, etc.

I.  Problems may arise when patients are on certain drugs.

J.  *Never* leave *any* patient unattended. There must *always* be a staff member in the room where the patient is being treated.

K.  Some treatments will require you to remain at the patient's side due to the nature of the modality or to the danger of leaving the patient alone.

L.  Protect yourself by using good body mechanics, by avoiding lifting unless absolutely necessary, etc.

M.  Personal liability insurance is an *excellent* investment.

## VI. Physical Therapy Records

A.  Adequate and precise information is important.

B.  The hospital and/or department procedures will determine the content.

| NAME_____ AGE____ PHYSICIAN_____ |
| ADDRESS_____ |
| DIAGNOSIS_____ |
| PRESCRIPTION_____ |

DAILY_____            BID_____            TID_____

|      | 1 | 2 | 3 | 4 | 5 | 6 | 7 | 8 | 9 | 10 | 11 | 12 | 13 | 14 | 15 | 16 | 17 | 18 | 19 | 20 | 21 | 22 | 23 | 24 | 25 | 26 | 27 | 28 | 29 | 30 | 31 |
|------|---|---|---|---|---|---|---|---|---|----|----|----|----|----|----|----|----|----|----|----|----|----|----|----|----|----|----|----|----|----|----|
| JAN  |   |   |   |   |   |   |   |   |   |    |    |    |    |    |    |    |    |    |    |    |    |    |    |    |    |    |    |    |    |    |    |
| FEB  |   |   |   |   |   |   |   |   |   |    |    |    |    |    |    |    |    |    |    |    |    |    |    |    |    |    |    |    |    |    |    |
| MAR  |   |   |   |   |   |   |   |   |   |    |    |    |    |    |    |    |    |    |    |    |    |    |    |    |    |    |    |    |    |    |    |
| APR  |   |   |   |   |   |   |   |   |   |    |    |    |    |    |    |    |    |    |    |    |    |    |    |    |    |    |    |    |    |    |    |
| MAY  |   |   |   |   |   |   |   |   |   |    |    |    |    |    |    |    |    |    |    |    |    |    |    |    |    |    |    |    |    |    |    |
| JUNE |   |   |   |   |   |   |   |   |   |    |    |    |    |    |    |    |    |    |    |    |    |    |    |    |    |    |    |    |    |    |    |
| JULY |   |   |   |   |   |   |   |   |   |    |    |    |    |    |    |    |    |    |    |    |    |    |    |    |    |    |    |    |    |    |    |
| AUG  |   |   |   |   |   |   |   |   |   |    |    |    |    |    |    |    |    |    |    |    |    |    |    |    |    |    |    |    |    |    |    |
| SEPT |   |   |   |   |   |   |   |   |   |    |    |    |    |    |    |    |    |    |    |    |    |    |    |    |    |    |    |    |    |    |    |
| OCT  |   |   |   |   |   |   |   |   |   |    |    |    |    |    |    |    |    |    |    |    |    |    |    |    |    |    |    |    |    |    |    |
| NOV  |   |   |   |   |   |   |   |   |   |    |    |    |    |    |    |    |    |    |    |    |    |    |    |    |    |    |    |    |    |    |    |
| DEC  |   |   |   |   |   |   |   |   |   |    |    |    |    |    |    |    |    |    |    |    |    |    |    |    |    |    |    |    |    |    |    |

Figure 6. Sample physical therapy treatment record.

```
┌─────────────────────────────────────────────────────────┐
│                    PROGRESS  NOTES                        │
│                                                           │
│                                                           │
│                                                           │
│                                                           │
│                                                           │
│                                                           │
│                                                           │
│                                                           │
│                                                           │
│                                                           │
│                                                           │
│                                                           │
└─────────────────────────────────────────────────────────┘
```

Figure 7. Sample physical therapy treatment record, reverse side.

C.   Adequate records should include:
   1. Inpatients:
      a. Patient's name.
      b. Marital status.
      c. Sex.
      d. Age.
      e. Room number.
      f. Diagnosis with physician's signature.
      g. Physician.
      h. Prescription.
      i. Date of treatment.
      j. Exact treatment given.
      k. Patient's comments as to how he is progressing, whether or not the treatment is helping, etc.
      l. Your notes regarding the patient's progress.
      m. The frequency of writing progress notes is determined by the patient's condition, the department policy, the therapist, and the physican.
   2. Outpatients:

a. Patient's name.
b. Marital status.
c. Sex.
d. Age.
e. Address.
f. Phone number.
g. Diagnosis with physician's signature.
h. Physician.
i. Prescription.
j. Date of treatment.
k. Exact treatment given.
l. Patient's comments.
m. Progress notes.
n. Billing for treatment to whom.

## VII. Prescriptions

A. In many cases, the qualified physical therapist will pre-
   scribe the treatment. Therefore, the responsibility rests with
   the therapist, and he must be fully aware of the dangers of
   using the wrong modality.
B. A good prescription should include:
   1. Patient's name.
   2. Sex.
   3. Diagnosis.
   4. Type of treatment.
   5. Areas to be treated.
   6. Frequency of treatment both per day and per week.
   7. Age.
   8. Precautions such as recent surgery; cardiac problems;
      implants both metal and electrical; speech, hearing,
      visual, or language problems; respiratory problems;
      drug sensitivity; psychiatric or retardation problems,
      etc.
   9. Special instructions such as do not remove the splint or
      brace; give the patient home instructions, etc.
   10. Signature of physician or physical therapist. If the
       order is called in, the signature should be obtained at a
       later date.

# Part II
# Superficial Heating Techniques

*Chapter 2*

# WARM WHIRLPOOL

## *I. Preparations*

A.  Determine the procedure to be used:
    1.  Select the correct size whirlpool if available.

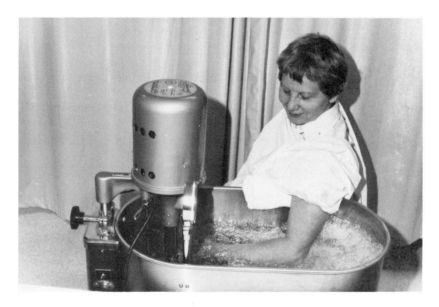

Figure 8. Arm whirlpool. (Ille Division of Market Forge.)

    2.  Select the most comfortable position for the patient.
    3.  The room temperature should be warm, no less than 80° F.

B.  Fill the clean whirlpool approximately two-thirds full of water:
    1.  Close the whirlpool drain and turn on the water.
    2.  Adjust the mixing valve to obtain water at the correct

31

temperature:
   a. Arm whirlpool — 102° F.
   b. Leg whirlpool — 100° F.
   c. Body whirlpool — 96° F.
   3. Do not overfill the tank:
      a. Some older tanks do not have overflow drains.
      b. If the tank is too full, placing the part/body into the water and/or action of the turbine will cause the water to overflow.
C. Add disinfectant if necessary:
   1. A disinfectant should be added to the water when treating infected or open lesions.
   2. A disinfectant may be used as a psychological aid.
   3. Disposable plastic liners may be used with proper agitation equipment.
D. Check the turbine:
   1. The turbine *must* be grounded.
   2. The line cord must be in excellent condition, and the plug should fit securely in the socket.
   3. Be *sure* that your hands are dry and that you are not standing in any water.
   4. Check to be *sure* the water intakes are completely covered with water.
   5. Check to be *sure* the turbine motor air intakes are uncovered.
   6. Turn on the turbine.
   7. Adjust the water pressure and air bubbles to the desired flow.
   8. Adjust the direction of the water flow.
   9. Turn off the turbine.
E. Have all other necessary materials ready to use:
   1. Turkish towels for drying and padding should be ready.
   2. Cephalic cold and tepid drinking water should be readily available.
   3. If the patient is to sit in the tank, appropriate clothing will be necessary.
   4. Whirlpool chair and/or stool castors should be locked

in place.

5. Drain and turbine strainers should be used if patches of dead skin and tissue will slough off during the treatment.

## II. *Starting the Treatment*

A. *Never* leave children, the elderly, psychotic, or retarded patients unattended.
B. Be *sure* there is no water on the floor.
C. Explain the procedure to the patient:
    1. Tell him the water is warm, and let him feel it.
    2. Explain the action of the turbine. Show him there is no propeller or anything that can hurt him.
    3. Instruct him not to cover the water intakes or outlets on the turbine, and tell him why.
    4. Caution him *never* to touch any switches (including the turbine switch), the conducting cord, or any electrical outlets.
    5. Demonstrate any exercises you want him to do while he is in the water.
D. Have the patient remove his clothing as necessary, and provide him with a T-binder, gown, bathing suit or other appropriate clothing.
    1. If treating the upper extremity, have the patient remove his shirt, dress, or blouse to prevent them from becoming wrinkled or wet from perspiration or the water. Do *not* allow the patient to roll up his sleeve, as this can impair circulation.
    2. If treating the lower extremity, have the patient remove trousers or slacks as well as shoes and socks. Do not allow the patient to roll up a pant leg.
    3. Provide the patient with cotton or paper scuffers to wear to and from the treatment area.
E. If one foot (ankle) is to be treated, do not treat both. Provide a footstool, or instruct the patient to put the non-treated foot on the rung of the whirlpool chair.
F. Have the patient remove his watch if treating the appro-

priate upper extremity or if the patient sits in the tank.
G. Remove all bandages, tapes, dressings, etc.:
   1. These will damage an operating turbine.
   2. Do *not* pull off dressings that stick. Allow them to soak in the water with the turbine off.
H. Unless contraindicated, remove all braces, splints, etc., so the patient may exercise in the water.
I. Check the area to be treated:
   1. Check for any unusual marks, open or infected lesions, edema, etc.
   2. If there is a skin rash, the patient must be medically cleared for treatment.
   3. Check skin sensation.
J. Recheck the water temperature both by the thermometer and by immersing your hand into the water.
K. Position the patient as necessary:
   1. Recheck to be sure all chair/stool castors are locked.
   2. If the patient is sitting outside the tank, pressure points caused by the edge of the tank should be padded with substantial and soft padding. If using a folded towel, tell the patient not to allow the towel to touch the water as it will act as a sponge and then water will drip onto him.
   3. A footstool may be necessary.
   4. Whirlpool seat:
      a. Be sure the seat is at the correct height.
      b. The patient may use the seat to get in and out of the tank as well as sit on it, or he may rest his foot/feet on it. Some seats must be held in place until the patient's weight is on them or they will float off of their holders.
L. Position the turbine:
   1. It may be desirable to direct the water and air stream away from the part because of the diagnosis or for the first few treatments.
   2. Adjust the depth of the turbine in the water. When raising the turbine, do not pull it off its holder.
M. Be sure your hands are dry and that you are not standing in

any water. Turn on the turbine.

N. If patches of dead skin slough off such as will happen when treating burns, frostbite or after long immobilization in a cast, turn off the turbine several times during the treatment, remove the skin and clean the turbine and drain cleaners.

O. Check the patient several times during the first treatment. During subsequent treatments, check him at least once during the treatment.

P. If the patient's face becomes flushed, use cephalic cold and offer him cool or tepid (not cold) water to drink.

Q. Treatment time is usually twenty to thirty minutes.

### III. Terminating the Treatment

A. Turn off the turbine and move it to one side.

B. Remove the extremity or patient from the water, and be sure he dries himself thoroughly.

C. Keep the patient warm.

D. Inspect the skin.

E. Empty and clean the tank and turbine. Use Bon Ami® or some other nonabrasive cleaner.

F. The possibility of cross-infection must be considered:
   1. If the patient has had an infected lesion or if you have an infected or open lesion on your hands, wear rubber gloves and use a disinfectant when cleaning the tank.
   2. After removing the gloves, do *not* touch your eyes, ears, nose or mouth until you have thoroughly washed your hands.

### IV. Notes

A. The whirlpool thermometers should be calibrated at least once a year depending on the amount of tank usage.

B. Swab procedure:
   1. This should be done at least once a month or as is indicated.
   2. When treating open, infected and/or draining lesions,

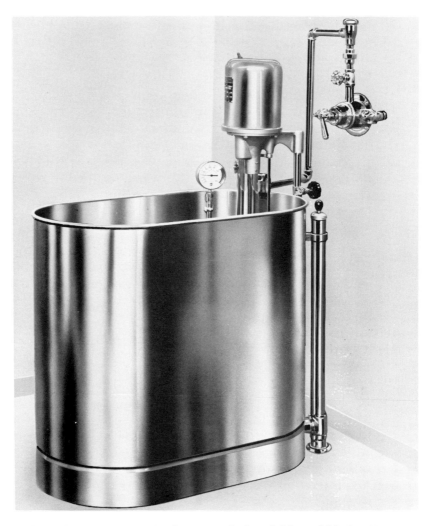

Figure 9. Leg whirlpool. (Courtesy of Ille Division of Market Forge.)

burns, etc., the swab procedure should be done at least once a day.
3. Check with the chief of the laboratory in your facility to find out the preferred procedure.
4. One method is to take a Q-tips® stick swab and run it around the inside of the water intake tube once. Imme-

diately place it into a sterile container, cover it, and take it to the laboratory.

    5. The whirlpool drain should be checked also.

C. To sterilize a whirlpool tank:

    1. Completely drain the tank.

    2. Scrub the tank, turbine and any equipment used in the tank with a brush and a disinfectant.

    3. Leave the equipment in the tank.

    4. Refill the tank with water at least 115° F.

    5. Depending on the size of the tank, aid at least 4 ounces of a strong disinfectant.

    6. Use a long handled brush to wash the tank sides, turbine tubes and other surfaces for five minutes while running.

    7. Turn off the turbine and wash the underside and up into the turbine tubes.

    8. Drain the tank, but leave any equipment on the bottom.

    9. Refill with water as hot as possible.

    10. Let it stand for at least five minutes.

    11. Add cold water or let the hot water cool sufficiently long enough to allow you to put your hand into it.

    12. Rinse the sides of the tank and equipment with a sponge.

    13. Drain the tank.

    14. Remove all equipment.

    15. Soak a sponge with the disinfectant and scrub the sides and bottom of the tank, turbine tubes and drains.

    16. Allow the tank to dry for at least thirty minutes before refilling.

## Chapter 3

# HYDROCOLLATOR® HOT PACKS

## *I. Preparations*

A. Determine the procedure to be used:
   1. Select the technique:
      a. Two-towel wrap.
      b. One-towel wrap.
      c. Unwrapped pack.

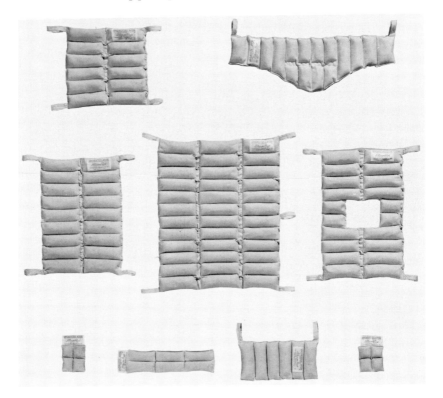

Figure 10. Hydrocollator steam packs. (Courtesy of Chattanooga Pharmacal Co.)

B. Check the unit:
    1. The unit must be grounded.
    2. The water should be clean and hot, 150° to 170° F. Use a candy or dairy thermometer to check the temperature. Do *not* put your hand into the water.
    3. The water should cover the packs at all times. If water has to be added, add it at the end of the day.

C. Check the packs:
    1. The proper size and shape packs should be ready to use.
    2. The pack should be thoroughly soaked. New packs should soak overnight.
    3. The pack seams should be intact. After prolonged use or soaking, the stitching may rot. Do not use brittle or old packs.
    4. The pack should be hot:
        a. Department routine may place the cold packs in the rear (front) of the unit.
        b. Allow from twenty to thirty minutes for the pack to reheat between patients if the water temperature is at least 150° F. A higher water temperature will heat a cold pack in ten to fifteen minutes.

D. Have all other necessary materials ready to use:
    1. Tongs will be needed for removing the pack that is completely covered with water:
        a. Take hold of the pack tabs with the tongs. Do *not* grasp the pack itself as the covering could be torn.
    2. *Do not put your hand into the water.* If the pack tabs are out of the water, you can take hold of the tabs with your fingers to remove the pack, as the tabs will be cool.
    3. Towels and/or pack covers will be needed for pack padding and drying the patient.

## II. Starting the Treatment

A. Explain the procedure to the patient:
    1. Tell him that the heat from the pack should be

comfortably warm and not hot, and tell him why.

    2. Explain that it may take several minutes for him to feel the warmth (depending on the amount of padding and the temperature of the pack).

    3. Impress him with the importance of calling you *immediately* if the packs are too hot or too heavy.

    4. If he becomes uncomfortable for any reason, he should call you *before* he moves as unwrapped packs can cause burns.

    5. Tell him his skin will be red after treatment.

B.  Use caution. A pack is very hot and heavy and the patient can be easily burned:

    1. The temperature must *always* be comfortable.

    2. Check the skin often. If it is bright red, add more toweling between the pack and the skin regardless of what the patient says about the heat.

    3. Be especially careful when treating the elderly and the very young.

C.  Check the area to be treated:

    1. Check skin sensation. If sensation is lacking or diminished, use *extreme* caution.

    2. Be careful to check for any unusual marks.

    3. Do *not* treat on new skin or recent scar tissue.

    4. If the area is painful to pressure, do *not* use a canvas covered pack unless it is very small. Instant hot packs or a whirlpool would be preferable.

D.  Do *not* allow the patient to lie on the pack:

    1. This can become very uncomfortable.

    2. The skin will become hot very quickly.

    3. With the use of extra pillows for the patient's comfort and support, the neck, an upper or lower extremity may be placed on the pack. More pack padding will probably be necessary especially when the pack is under an extremity.

E.  Two-towel wrap:

    1. Take two large, heavy turkish towels (no hand towels), and fold each one lengthwise once.

    2. Place one towel on top of the other in the form of a

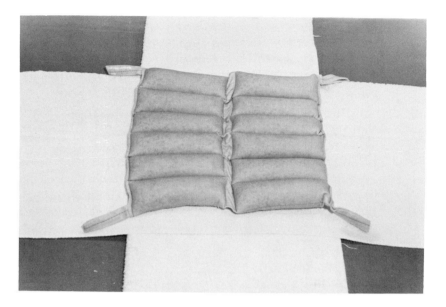

Figure 11. Two-towel wrap.

cross (+).

3. Remove the correct size heated pack from the unit.
4. Allow the excess water to drip into the tank. Do not "wave" the pack in the air, as this hastens the cooling process.
5. Place the pack on the center of the crossed towels. (If more than one pack is to be used, wrap each pack separately.)
6. Do not bother to fold in the pack tabs. They do not contain any silica gel and therefore no heat.
7. Fold the ends of the towels over the pack. This will result in eight layers of toweling on top of the pack.
8. Close the unit lid.
9. Warn the patient and place the pack on the area to be treated with the eight layers of toweling next to the skin.

F. One-towel wrap (used when the pack is too large to wrap as above):

1. Take three heavy turkish towels and fold each one in half once.
2. Lay each folded towel on top of the other, resulting in six layers of toweling.
3. Place the three folded towels on the area to be treated.
4. Remove the correct size heated pack from the unit. Do not "wave" the pack in the air as this hastens the cooling.
5. Allow the excess water to drip into the tank.
6. Wrap the entire pack in a heavy turkish towel being sure no part of the pack is exposed.
7. Place the thinly wrapped side of the pack on the towels on the patient.
8. Cover the pack with another turkish towel to slow the loss of heat.
9. Close the unit lid.

G. Unwrapped pack:
1. Take four heavy turkish towels and fold each one in half.
2. Lay each towel on top of the other resulting in eight layers of toweling.
3. Place all four towels on the area to be treated.
4. Remove the correct size heated pack from the unit. Do not "wave" the pack in the air, as this hastens the heat loss.
5. Allow the excess water to drip into the tank.
6. Place the pack on the towels on the patient.
7. Cover the pack with one turkish towel folded in half to retard the heat loss.
8. Close the unit lid.

H. Oddly shaped packs such as a neck pack should be wrapped so there will be six to eight layers of toweling between the pack and the skin.

I. Hold the packs in place with towels, sheets, light sandbags or straps. It is always preferable to place the pack on the patient rather than placing the patient on the pack.

J. Commercial pack covers may be used:
1. Several layers of heavy turkish toweling may have to be

added between the pack cover and the skin for insulation.

    2. If pack covers are to be used on several patients between washings:

        a. At least one layer of toweling should be used between the pack cover and skin for hygienic purposes.

        b. The pack covers should always be dried before they are used again.

K. *No part of an unwrapped pack should ever touch the patient.*

L. Check the skin after a few minutes:

    1. More layers of toweling may be needed no matter what the technique.

    2. If less toweling is needed after a few minutes of treatment, either the pack did not have sufficient time to reheat between patients or the unit water was not hot enough.

M. Do *not* remove toweling or change the packs as they begin to cool.

N. Do *not* use an infrared lamp over a pack to keep it hot.

O. Do *not* use another modality on the *same* patient at the same time you are using hot packs. Use each modality separately.

P. Treatment time is usually twenty to thirty minutes.

### III. Terminating the Treatment

A. Remove the pack and toweling from the patient.

B. Check the skin for any unusual marks that were not there before treatment.

C. Give the patient a dry turkish towel and instruct (help) him to dry himself thoroughly.

D. Suggest to the patient that he wait in the reception area for a few minutes to cool off before going outside.

E. Place the packs in the designated area in the unit.

F. Close the unit lid.

G. Dispose of any toweling used next to the patient. It should be dried as much as possible before being placed in the laundry basket.

H.  Hang or spread the other towels to dry. Do *not* use wet or damp towels on the next patient.

## IV. Notes

A.  Do *not* allow the packs to dry out as they will become hard and brittle. If they are used only occasionally, unplug the unit line cord but leave the packs in the water.

B.  Allow the water and packs to heat overnight when activating a new unit or one that has not been used for some time.

C.  The unit water should be changed once a month depending on usage.

D.  The unit should be cleaned once a month depending on

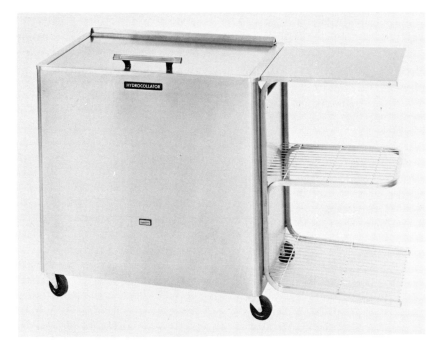

Figure 12. Hydrocollator steam pack heating unit. (Courtesy of Chattanooga Pharmacal Co.)

usage:
1. Drain the tank.
2. Clean the tank and pack rack using a mild disinfectant, soap and hot water. Do not use abrasives.
E. Home use of commercial packs:
1. The standard size commercial pack may be purchased for ten dollars.
2. Instruct the patient in the correct use of the pack, and have him practice in the department before using the pack at home:
   a. If the pack has never been used, hold it by the tabs with the sections in a horizontal position, and shake the pack gently to distribute the gel filler.
   b. Place the pack in a container large enough to accommodate the pack when it is completely covered with water, and a container that can be heated such as a stainless steel roasting pan or kettle. Do not use an aluminum container as the packs can be stained.
   c. Fill the container with enough water to cover the pack, and allow it to soak for several hours.
   d. After the pack is thoroughly wet, place the container on the stove and bring the water to a boil.
   e. Reduce the heat control to low, and allow the pack to heat for thirty minutes.
   f. Prepare the heavy turkish towels. The two-towel wrap is the safest method.
   g. Using a fork or pliers, take hold of a corner loop and remove the pack from the water.
   h. Allow the excess water to drip into the container or sink. Tell the patient not to "wave" the pack in the air.
   i. Place the pack on the crossed towels, and fold the ends over the pack.
   j. Place the pack on the area to be treated, and leave the pack in place for twenty to thirty minutes.
   k. If the heat is too intense, put one or two layers of turkish toweling between the pack and skin.
   l. Do *not* remove toweling or replace the pack as it

cools.

3. The patient should be told how many times a day/week to use the pack.
4. Care of the pack:
   a. The pack should be kept in water if it is to be used frequently.
   b. When the pack is no longer needed, tightly seal the cooled *wet* pack in a plastic bag, and store it in a refrigerator or freezer; the pack should not be allowed to dry out.

*Chapter 4*

# INSTANT HOT PACKS

## *I. Preparations*

A. Determine the procedure to be used:
   1. Patient's position for treatment.
   2. Know how to use the pack:
      a. Some packs must be soaked in hot water for five minutes, and they are reusable. (The water in a hot pack commercial unit may be used to soak the pack.)
      b. Other packs are activated by breaking/shaking the bag to mix the contents. These must be disposed of after using once. This type of pack is not recommended for the physical therapy department as it can become expensive.
B. Have all necessary materials ready to use:
   1. Turkish towels will be needed for padding.
   2. Tongs should be used to remove packs from the water.

## *II. Starting the Treatment*

A. Explain the treatment procedure to the patient:
   1. Tell him the heat from the packs should be comfortably warm and not hot, and tell him why.
   2. Explain that it may take several minutes for him to feel the warmth.
   3. Tell him to call you *immediately* if the packs are too hot or heavy.
   4. If he becomes uncomfortable for any reason, he should call you *before* he moves as an unwrapped pack can cause burns.
   5. Tell him his skin will be red after treatment.
B. Use caution:
   1. The temperature must *always* be comfortable.

2. If the skin is bright red, add more toweling between the pack and skin regardless of what the patient says about the heat.

C. Check the area to be treated:
   1. Check the skin sensation. If sensation is lacking or diminished, use caution.
   2. Check for any unusual marks on the skin.
   3. Do *not* treat on new skin or recent scar tissue.

D. Do *not* allow the patient to lie on the pack:
   1. This can become very uncomfortable.
   2. The skin will become hot very quickly.
   3. There is always the possibility the pack cover may rupture. Therefore, this practice is highly discouraged.

E. Place one layer of turkish toweling on the skin.

F. Activate the pack/remove it from the water.

G. Place the pack on the towel.

H. Cover the pack with the towel or another towel.

I. Hold the pack in place with a light sandbag or the pack towel.

J. Check the skin after a few minutes.

K. Do *not* remove toweling or change the pack as it begins to cool.

L. Do *not* use an infrared lamp over the pack to keep it warm.

M. Do *not* use another modality on the same patient at the same time you are treating with a pack.

N. Treatment time is about ten minutes.

### III. Terminating the Treatment

A. Remove the pack and toweling.

B. Check the skin for any unusual marks or erythema.

### IV. Home Use of Instant Packs

A. The patient should be thoroughly instructed in the use of the pack.

B. The patient should practice the technique several times in the department.

C. Warn the patient of the dangers.
D. Give him written directions and list the dangers.
E. Tell him how many times to use the packs each day.

*Chapter 5*

# MELTED PARAFFIN

## *I. Preparations*

A.  Determine the procedure to be used:
    1. Paraffin dip. This technique must be used on the extremities when the demand for paraffin treatments does not allow time for the immersion technique to be used on each patient.
    2. Paraffin immersion. This technique is used on the extremities and produces greater heating effects than does the dip technique.
    3. The paraffin painting technique is used when other forms of heat are not available or to treat parts of the body that cannot be treated by the first two methods.
    4. The paraffin wrap technique is not used much because it wastes paraffin.
    5. The paraffin pouring technique is used only when the part cannot be dipped or immersed or when other forms of heat are not available.
B.  Select the unit to be used:
    1. If hands and feet are treated in the department, two baths should be available.
    2. Baths vary in size and shape according to the manufacturer.
C.  Check the paraffin mixture temperature:
    1. After the paraffin is melted, it will take from three to four hours (depending on the size of the unit) for the paraffin and oil to cool to the treatment temperature of between 126° and 130° F.
    2. Once the mixture is at the correct temperature, a thermostat maintains that temperature.
    3. Use a candy or dairy thermometer, and leave it in the mixture for several minutes.

50

    4. Do *not* use the paraffin bath if the temperature exceeds 130° F or is lower than 126° F. To lower the temperature, remove the unit lid, unplug the line cord or readjust the thermostat.

D. Have all materials ready to use:
    1. Wax paper, aluminum foil, plastic sheets or bags or paper towels will be needed for initial wrapping.
    2. Turkish towels may be used for the second wrapping.
    3. Masking tape should be ready to secure the toweling.

E. Place the chair or plinth in such a position that the patient and you have easy access to the paraffin. Avoid moving the paraffin bath if possible.

F. Protect the floor around the unit from any spilled paraffin:
    1. If paraffin drips onto the floor, etc., allow it to harden and then scrape it up.
    2. Even after scraping up the paraffin, the floor may be very slippery.

## II. Starting the Treatment

A. Explain the procedure to the patient:
    1. Tell him the paraffin will feel hot, but it will not burn him. Demonstrate on yourself if necessary.
    2. Caution him about touching the insides of the unit. The bottom is usually protected by slats.
    3. Tell him why the treatment is being done and what it will do for him.
    4. Tell him his skin may be red after treatment.

B. Inspect the part to be treated:
    1. Remove watches and rings if in the treatment area. If rings cannot be removed, cover them with several thicknesses of gauze, and hold the gauze in place with masking tape.
    2. The skin must be clean in order not to contaminate the mixture. It is always a good procedure to have (help) the patient wash with soap and water to remove any perspiration and dead skin.
    3. The skin must be dry as perspiration or water droplets

        can cause burns.

    4. Any open or draining lesions, rashes, infections, new skin or recent scar tissue are contraindications for treatment.

C. Check skin sensation. If sensation is lacking or diminished, use paraffin with caution.

D. Position the patient properly and drape him if appropriate:

    1. If the patient's hand/forearm are to be treated:

        a. Place the patient at the side of the tank.

        b. Be sure his feet will rest comfortably on the floor if treating his hand, etc.

        c. Place a turkish towel on his lap.

        d. On the towel, place wax paper, paper towels, etc. in which to wrap the extremity.

        e. If the immersion technique is to be used, the edge of the tank may have to be padded.

    2. If the patient's feet/ankles are to be treated:

        a. The patient may sit on the end/side of a plinth. If possible, take the plinth to the paraffin bath instead of taking the bath to the plinth.

        b. If using the immersion technique, the edge of the tank may have to be padded.

E. Be sure the patient's clothing is protected from the paraffin.

F. Paraffin dip:

    1. The patient's fingers (toes) should be relaxed. This is especially important when treating the hand. The tendency will be for the patient to extend the fingers and thumb. It will be impossible for him to keep them extended for twenty minutes. When he relaxes his fingers, cracks may occur in the paraffin glove allowing the part to cool faster.

    2. The wrist should be at $0°$.

    3. Remove the unit lid.

    4. Instruct (help) the patient to dip the part into the paraffin mixture.

    5. As soon as the part is covered with paraffin (a few seconds), remove it from the bath.

    6. The patient must not move his fingers (toes), etc.

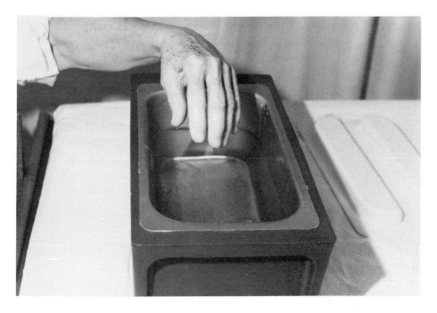

Figure 13. Paraffin dip. (Parabath by Talcott Laboratories.)

7. Hold the part over the tank allowing the excess paraffin to drip off.
8. As soon as the paraffin has solidified and lost its shiny appearance (five seconds or less), the part should be dipped again.
9. Repeat the dipping procedure six to twelve times. Dip to the *same* level each time or to below the level of the first dip.
10. After the final dip, quickly place the paper towels or waxed paper around the final layer being sure to cover all surfaces.
11. Wrap the part neatly in a turkish towel to further retard the cooling process. Make sure the toweling is fitted tightly around the wrist (ankle).
12. Use masking tape to hold the toweling in place.
13. Close the unit lid.
14. The treatment time is twenty to thirty minutes.

G. Paraffin immersion:
1. Repeat the above dipping procedure six to twelve

times.

2. After the final removal, allow the paraffin to solidify.
3. Place the part back into the paraffin.
4. Leave the part in the tank from twenty to thirty minutes or until the paraffin melts. Be sure the patient is in a comfortable position. Padding the edge of the tank will aid in comfort.

H. Paraffin painting:
1. Protect any clothing, linens and floor area from the paraffin.
2. Warn the patient that you are going to apply the paraffin.
3. Using any ordinary paint brush, dip it into the paraffin.
4. Remove the brush and immediately brush on the paraffin to the area that cannot be dipped.
5. Allow the first layer to solidify and lose its shiny appearance.
6. Repeat six to twelve times. Do not allow the paraffin to drip onto another part of the patient.
7. Cover the paraffin with paper towels or wax paper.
8. Cover the paper towels with a turkish towel to reduce cooling.
9. Close the unit lid.
10. Caution the patient about moving.
11. Leave in place twenty to thirty minutes.

I. Paraffin wrap:
1. Dip the part once (or paint on one layer of paraffin).
2. Cover the first layer with one thickness of gauze.
3. Repeat this process six to twelve times.
4. After the final layer of gauze, wrap or cover the part with paper towels or wax paper.
5. Cover the paper towels with a turkish towel.
6. Close the unit lid.
7. Leave in place twenty to thirty minutes.
8. This is a rather wasteful method as it is difficult to save the paraffin.

J. Paraffin pouring:

1. Protect any clothing and the floor from paraffin.
2. Hold the part over the tank if possible.
3. Using a cup, pour the paraffin onto the part to be treated, reaching all surfaces.
4. Allow the paraffin to solidify.
5. Repeat six to twelve times.
6. Cover or wrap as above.
7. Close the unit lid.
8. Leave in place for twenty to thirty minutes.

## III. Terminating the Treatment

A. Remove the wrappings.
B. Peel off the paraffin.
C. Spread out the paraffin as much as possible, and replace it in the tank. The paraffin will melt faster if spread out instead of being wadded up. (Ideally, used paraffin should be discarded, but this can prove to be very costly.)
D. Close unit lid.
E. Have the patient wipe himself off.
F. Check the patient's skin.

## IV. Notes

A. A desirable commercial unit should include:
   1. Insulation.
   2. Slats on the inside bottom of the tank.
   3. Thermostatic control.
   4. Thermometer.
   5. Timer:
      a. The timer is *not* a treatment timer.
      b. When the timer is turned on, it *deactivates* the thermostat allowing the temperature of the paraffin to rise to between 180° and 200° F depending on the time set.
      c. This high temperature allows sterilization of the tank.
B. Care of the equipment (Thermo-Electric Corporation):

1. Most paraffin baths should be sterilized once a month depending on usage.
2. Units should be cleaned regularly to remove the moisture and sediment that collect at the bottom:
   a. Paraffin should be liquid.
   b. Unplug the line cord.
   c. Dip out the paraffin into another large container down to the slats.
   d. Remove and clean the slats:
      1. Allow the paraffin to solidify.
      2. Scrape off as much paraffin as possible.
      3. Dispose of this paraffin.
      4. Wash the slats in hot soap and water.
   e. Dip out and dispose of the paraffin remaining in the bottom of the tank. Use paper towels to remove the dregs; do *not* attempt to pour out the paraffin.
   f. Replace the slats and paraffin mixture.
C. Alternate cleaning method:
   1. Leave the unit plugged into the outlet.
   2. Place six teaspoons of boric acid powder into one gallon of hot water (large tanks).
   3. Pour this into the bath mixture. It will flow to the bottom of the tank. Some paraffin will congeal unless the water and boric acid mixture is extremely hot.
   4. Allow the boric acid mixture to flow to the drain end of the unit.
   5. Open the drain by turning the drain handle on the bottom of the tank six full turns.
   6. Press the drain switch button on the control panel until the mixture begins to flow.
   7. As soon as the solution starts to flow, release the drain switch button.
   8. Allow all of the water and some of the paraffin to drain.
   9. Push the drain switch button and close the drain.
D. Home use of paraffin:
   1. Paraffin is *very* flammable. Caution the patient about keeping the paraffin away from an open flame.

2. A double boiler *must* be used.
3. Heat the paraffin and oil in the top of a double boiler until the paraffin is melted. The ratio of mineral oil to paraffin is 1/2 to 1 ounce of oil to 1 pound of paraffin.
4. Cool the mixture until a thin coating forms on the top.
5. Check the temperature of the mixture using a dairy or candy thermometer. The temperature should not exceed 130° F.
6. Instruct the patient:
   a. How to do the dip or immersion procedure.
   b. How long the paraffin should remain on the part.
   c. How many times a day to use the treatment.
   d. The part must be dry before using the paraffin.
   e. How to clean up any spilled paraffin.

## Chapter 6

# INFRARED RADIATION

## Luminous and Nonluminous Lamps

### *I. Preparations*

A. Select the generator:
   1. The choice of a luminous or nonluminous generator usually depends on what is available. If both are available, luminous radiation penetrates deeper than does nonluminous radiation.
   2. Select the correct size lamp if available.
   3. Make *sure* you have selected an infrared lamp and not an ultraviolet lamp.
B. Check the lamp:
   1. Know how to operate the lamp and the manual adjustments.
   2. The lamp should be grounded.
   3. The lamp reflector (and tube in the luminous quartz lamps) should be clean and dust free. Use Bon Ami, absolute alcohol or distilled water and a soft cloth.
   4. Be sure the lamp is operating safely and efficiently:
      a. All manual adjustments *must* be in working order.
      b. Do *not* use the lamp if the line cord is frayed.
      c. All plug and wire connections should be tight.
      d. Tubes, cores, bulbs, etc. should be secure.
      e. The screen or protective grid should be secure.
C. Turn on the nonluminous lamp to heat for five to ten minutes:
   1. If you are using a combination infrared and ultraviolet lamp, make *certain* you have turned on the infrared and *not* the ultraviolet.
D. Put the lamp at the back of the treatment booth out of the patient's way.

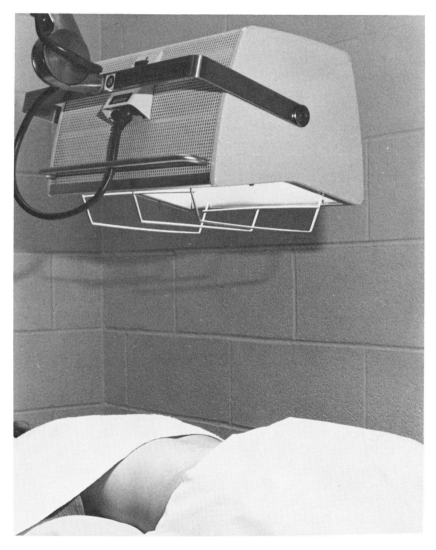

Figure 14. Infrared lamp. (Burkick Corp.)

E. Have all other materials ready to use.

## II. Starting the Treatment

A. Explain the procedure to the patient:

1. Tell him what to expect.
2. Explain the sensation he should feel:
   a. Tell him the heat should feel comfortably warm and *not* hot, and tell him why.
   b. Tell him he should call you *immediately* if the heat is too intense.
3. Caution him about touching the line cord, adjustments or any part of the lamp reflector.
4. Tell him his skin will be red and blotchy after the treatment, but it will disappear after a few minutes.

B.  Place the patient in the correct position. Instruct him not to move as he could be burned.
C.  Be sure the patient is properly draped.
D.  Check the area to be treated:
   1. The skin should be clean and free from oils, lotions and creams.
   2. All recent scar tissue, any abrasions or new skin should be covered with thick, wet pads of gauze or cotton. Hold the covering in place with masking tape.
   3. Cover (remove) any metal such as rings, earrings, etc. (if applicable) to prevent them from becoming hot and causing burns.
   4. Check skin sensation. If sensation is lacking or diminished, use caution. Check the skin often during treatment.
   5. If treating the face:
      a. Contact lenses should be removed.
      b. Cover the eyes with thick, wet pads of cotton or gauze.
   6. If treating the chest or a shoulder, the ears as well as the eyes may have to be protected.
E.  Position of the lamp:
   1. The distance between the lamp and the patient should be an estimated distance of at least 30 inches. If the distance is any less, the lamp will probably have to be raised after a few minutes because the heat will become

too intense. When raising or lowering the lamp, place your foot on the lamp base to hold it in place, and use the lamp adjustments. (Some old model lamps will separate in the middle when being raised, so use caution.)

2. The lamp should be centered both lengthways and sideways above the area to be treated.

3. The lamp reflector should be at a right angle to the skin.

F. Turn on the luminous lamp. (The nonluminous lamp should have been preheated.)

G. Remind the patient to call you *immediately* if the heat becomes too intense:

1. He should keep calling until someone comes.

2. It is your responsibility to drop whatever you are doing and go to the patient immediately.

H. To reduce the intensity, cover the part with one layer of the drape sheet or a light hand towel. (Covering the part changes the type of heat transfer from radiation to conduction.) Do not use a turkish towel, as it will take too long to heat.

I. Check back with the patient several times during the treatment. Add another layer of drape sheet any time the heat is too intense and/or when the skin is a bright, mottled red color.

J. The treatment time is usually twenty to thirty minutes.

### III. Terminating the Treatment

A. Turn off the lamp, unplug the line cord and drape it over the lamp arm once or use the hook provided on the lamp. (If using a nonluminous lamp and another patient is to follow within ten minutes, leave the lamp on to avoid the preheating time).

B. Move the lamp to the back of the booth out of the patient's way.

C. Warn the patient that the lamp is hot.

D. Give the patient a turkish towel, and tell him to dry his

skin if he has perspired.
E.  *Check the skin for any unusual marks that were not there before starting the treatment.*
F.  Suggest to the patient that he remain in the reception area for five to ten minutes to cool off before going outside.

## *IV. Notes*

A.  When moving lamps:
   1. Lower the lamp to lower the center of gravity.
   2. Retract large lamps.
   3. Watch for low doorways, curtain rods, etc.
B.  Check lamp castors occasionally for lint.

### BAKERS

## *I. Preparations*

A.  Bakers may be used to treat the extremities or the trunk.
B.  Determine the procedure to be used:
   1. Select the correct size baker.
   2. Select the patient's position in relation to his comfort and relaxation and whether or not the unit line cord will reach to the electrical outlet.
C.  Check the baker:
   1. The baker should be grounded.
   2. The line cord should not be frayed.
   3. The plug and wire connections should be tight.
   4. All bulbs should be working.
   5. Check to be sure all bulbs are secure.
   6. All manual adjustments *must* be in working order:
      a. The baker leg and folding manual adjustments should be checked *very* carefully.
D.  Have all materials ready to use:
   1. Cephalic cold should be readily available.
   2. Tepid drinking water should be ready.

3. Towels for reducing the heat intensity should be handy.

## II. Starting the Treatment

A. Explain the procedure to the patient:
  1. Tell him what you are going to do.
  2. Explain the sensation he *should* feel:
    a. Tell him that the heat should be comfortably warm and *not* hot, and tell him why.
    b. Tell him he should call you *immediately* if it is too hot or if he is uncomfortable for any reason.
    c. He should not move until you or someone has come.
  3. Caution him about touching the inside or outside of the baker, the adjustments or the line cord.
  4. Reassure him. Some patients may be apprehensive when under a full body baker.
B. If using a body or lower extremity baker, tell the patient to completely undress, and instruct him how to put on a T-binder or other appropriate clothing. Women should be provided with a towel to cover the breast area.
C. Place the patient in the correct position, and be sure he is properly draped.
D. Check the area to be treated:
  1. The skin should be clean and free from oils, creams, lotions, etc.
  2. All recent scar tissue, any abrasions or new skin should be covered with wet, thick pads of gauze or cotton. Hold the covering in place with masking tape.
  3. Cover (remove) any metal such as rings, bracelets, etc. (if applicable) to prevent them from becoming hot and causing burns.
  4. Check skin sensation. If sensation is lacking or diminished, check the skin often during the treatment.
E. Position the baker over the part to be treated:
  1. All baker adjustments should be made *before* positioning the baker over the patient.
  2. You may require assistance when lifting and posi-

tioning the baker due to its awkwardness.

3. *Never* carry the baker over the patient's head or face.
4. If possible, put the end of the baker to which the conducting cord is attached out of the patient's reach. This may necessitate the patient's head being toward the foot of the plinth.
5. Special attention must be given to the baker legs. The legs *must* be secure on the plinth. If the plinth has a ridge around the edge, all four baker legs must be *inside* of this ridge. If the plinth does not have a ridge around the edge, the legs *must* be secured with sandbags (not recommended).
6. *Never* raise or lower the baker while it is over the patient.
7. Be sure the patient's drape sheet is out from under the baker legs.

F. Methods of draping the baker:
   1. First method:
      a. Cover the entire baker and air spaces between the baker and the plinth/patient with a drape sheet.
      b. Ask the patient to hold onto the genital/breast draping.
      c. Go to the end of the baker next to the wall and lift the end of the baker drape sheet enough to grasp the patient's drape sheet.
      d. Remove the patient's drape sheet.
   2. Second method:
      a. Ask the patient to hold onto the genital/breast draping.
      b. From the curtain end of the booth, pull the patient's drape sheet off of him, and at the same time, slide it up on top of the baker. Avoid exposing the patient.
      c. Check to be sure all air spaces are closed.

G. If the patient's upper extremities are not to be treated, have him bring them outside of the baker drape sheet and cover them with another sheet or towels.

H. Turn on the desired number of bulbs. Usually all bulbs are turned on initially.

I. Remind the patient not to touch any part of the baker and not to move any part of his body covered by the baker drape sheet.

J. If the heat becomes too intense:
1. Make sure the genital/breast draping is in place, and then raise one or both ends of the baker drape sheet. Fold it up over the top of the baker, and/or
2. Turn off one or more sets of bulbs.

K. If the patient's face becomes flushed, apply cephalic cold and offer him tepid water to drink.

I. Treatment time is usually twenty to thirty minutes.

### III. Terminating the Treatment

A. Turn off all bulbs.
B. Remind the patient not to move as the baker will be very hot.
C. Redrape the patient:
1. First method:

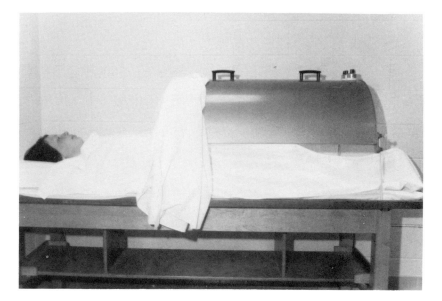

Figure 15. Lower extremity baker.

       a. Cover the patient with a drape sheet. He can assist you, but you must be sure he keeps his hands close to his body.

  2. Second method:

       a. Use the baker drape sheet. As you slide it off of the baker, pull it up over the patient. He may help you, but tell him to keep his hands close to his body. Be certain the patient remains properly draped.

D. Uncover the baker and if time allows, leave it over the patient for a few minutes to allow it to cool.

E. Unplug the line cord and wrap it around the baker handle.

F. Get someone to help you remove the baker if necessary. Do *not* take the baker over the patient's face or head.

G. Check the skin for any unusual marks that were not there before starting the treatment.

H. Ask the patient to remain in the waiting area for five to ten minutes to cool off before going outside.

## Chapter 7

# MOIST AIR

## *I. Preparations*

A. Determine the procedure to be used.
B. Select the patient's position:
    1. The patient is usually either supine or prone.
    2. Pillows should be used under the head and knees if the patient is supine.
    3. If the patient is prone, pillows should go under the low back and legs (do not include the knees or feet).
C. Check the unit:
    1. Know how to operate the unit.
    2. The unit must be grounded.
    3. Check the water level:
        a. The tank should be full.
        b. If water needs to be added, hot water will reduce heating time.
        c. When the tank is full, an amber light will glow and it will remain on until the unit is unplugged or if the tank needs water.
    4. Plug in the line cord.
    5. Set the intensity control to approximately 3. Experience will determine where the control must be set for the water temperature to reach and be maintained at 118° F.
    6. Push the reset button:
        a. If the red light comes on, the water heater is operating.
        b. Allow thirty to forty minutes for the water to reach a temperature of 118° F.
    7. The cabinet hood should be at the foot of the plinth.
    8. Wipe off any moisture on the inside of the hood.
    9. Do not cover the hood vents.

     10. Be sure the plinth extension is secure.

C.  Have all necessary materials ready to use:
  1. Appropriate clothing, T-binder, etc.
  2. Turkish towels.
  3. Bath blanket or drape sheet.
  4. Tepid drinking water and a straw.
  5. Cephalic cold should be readily available.
  6. Watch to time the patient's pulse.

## *II. Starting the Treatment*

A.  Recheck the unit temperature *before* placing the patient into the cabinet. If the temperature is over 120° F or under 115° F, do *not* treat the patient.

B.  Explain the procedure to the patient.
  1. Tell him that the hood will be over the part of his body that will be treated.
  2. Explain what the treatment will do.
  3. He will hear a noise that will be the vaporizer and fan.
  4. He should call you *immediately* if he is uncomfortable for any reason (too hot, dizzy, faint, nauseated, etc.).
  5. Explain what the treatment is.
  6. Tell him how long the treatment will be.
  7. Tell him he will hear a bell when the unit shuts off.

C.  The patient should evacuate bowels and bladder before starting the treatment.

D.  Have the patient completely undress, and give him a hospital gown, T-binder or other appropriate clothing. If only one-half of the body is to be treated, the patient should totally undress to prevent his underclothing from becoming wet from the moist air or perspiration. Provide draping for the breast and genital areas if necessary.

E.  Give the patient tepid water, and urge him to drink it. Explain to him that he will lose a lot of water through perspiration, especially if the whole body is being treated.

F.  Be *sure* the plinth extension is secure.

G.  Assist the patient onto the plinth, and position him comfortably.

H. Check the skin for any unusual marks.
I. Check skin sensation.
J. Cover the patient with a bath blanket or a sheet.
K. Slide the hood toward the patient's head until it is midway over his body or the part to be treated:
 1. The hood tracks must be free of linen.
 2. Make sure the patient's hands/elbows are not in the way.
L. If the entire body is to be treated:
 1. Drop the curtain at the head end of the hood.
 2. Place a turkish towel lengthwise across the patient's chest and shoulders for hygienic purposes and to absorb perspiration.
 3. Place the curtain on the towel, and tuck in the curtain and towel around the patient's neck and shoulders. Do not tuck them in too tightly around the patient's neck, but all air spaces must be closed.

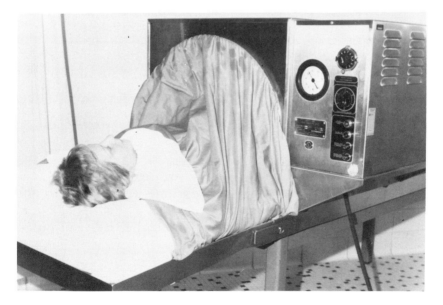

Figure 16. Moist air. (Ille Division of Market Forge.)

 4. Go to the foot end of the plinth and drop the curtain.
 5. Ask the patient to hold onto the breast/genital draping.

6. Lift the hood curtain only enough to remove the drape sheet or blanket.
7. Place a towel over the patient's feet, and tuck in the towel and curtain. Check to be sure all air spaces are closed.

M. If treating the upper half of the body:
   1. Follow the head end procedure as above.
   2. The foot end curtain should be tucked in over a towel around the patient's waist or at the level of the pelvis.
   3. Cover the patient's lower extremities with a bath blanket or drape sheet.

N. If treating the lower extremities:
   1. The head end curtain should be tucked in over a towel at either the patient's waist or at the level of the pelvis and the foot end curtain tucked in over a towel around his feet.
   2. Cover the upper half of the body with a bath blanket or drape sheet. Be sure the patient is warm.

O. *Before* turning on the unit, check the patient's pulse rate:
   1. *If the pulse rate is over 100 beats per minute, do not treat the patient.*
   2. Use the carotid or temporal arteries.
   3. Time the pulse rate for at least thirty seconds, using a watch with a second hand.
   4. The normal pulse rate for women is between 78 and 82 beats per minute, and that for men is between 70 and 72 beats per minute.

P. Set the unit timer to the desired treatment time:
   1. The unit is activated by the timer as indicated by the noise of the vaporizer and fan.
   2. The treatment time is usually twenty to thirty minutes.

Q. If the patient is apprehensive:
   1. Remain with him for the first few minutes or through the first treatment.
   2. Open the treatment cubicle curtains.
   3. Check back with him frequently.

R. *Check the patient's pulse occasionally.* If the pulse rate goes over 100 beats per minute at any time, terminate the treatment *immediately.*

S. If the patient's face becomes flushed:
   1. Use cephalic cold.
   2. Offer him tepid water to drink and urge him to drink it.

### III. Terminating the Treatment

A. The unit will be shut off by the timer:
   1. A bell will sound when the unit shuts off.
   2. If it is necessary to terminate treatment before the time is over, turn the time counterclockwise and the unit will shut off.
B. *Before* removing the hood curtains, drape the patient, preferably with a soft, absorbent bath blanket.
C. When the patient is completely draped, lift the cabinet curtains and drape them over the hood to dry.
D. Slide the cabinet to the foot end of the plinth.
E. Give the patient a turkish towel and have (help) him dry himself thoroughly.
F. Keep the patient draped, and have him sit on the side of the plinth for a few minutes before he stands:
   1. You should stand directly in front of him. However, be aware that he could fall backwards also.
   2. Check his pulse rate.
   3. Offer him water to drink.
   4. If he feels faint or dizzy, have him lie down for a few minutes and cool off.
G. Allow him to stand, and tell him to dress.
H. Suggest that he remain in the waiting room twenty minutes to cool off before going outside.

### IV. Notes

A. Lubrication (Market Forge): The motor should be lubricated every two or three months:
   1. Remove the louvre cover by taking out the three screws in the front and rear of each panel.

  2. Use only two drops of a lightweight, good grade motor oil in each cap.

B. Thermostat readjustment (Market Forge):
  1. Operate the unit with the heater on.
  2. Set the thermostat at 3 and allow the water to heat.
  3. Pull off the black plastic knob.
  4. Loosen, do *not* remove, the two round head screws.
  5. Hold onto the 1-inch diameter main body with two fingers of one hand.
  6. With the other hand, rotate the metal disc with the two elongated slots marked *L* and *R* clockwise to raise the temperature and counterclockwise to lower the temperature.
  7. Leave the screws loose and the knob off.
  8. Allow the heater to continue working for one hour.
  9. Check the thermometer.
  10. If the temperature is correct, replace the knob and tighten the screws.

C. The cabinet curtains will need washing in lukewarm water and a mild soap occasionally.

D. The cabinet mat should be washed once a month depending on usage:
  1. Use a mild antiseptic solution.
  2. Wash top, sides, ends and bottom of the mat.
  3. After cleaning, tip the mat on its side to allow it to dry.

# Part III
# Deep Heating Techniques

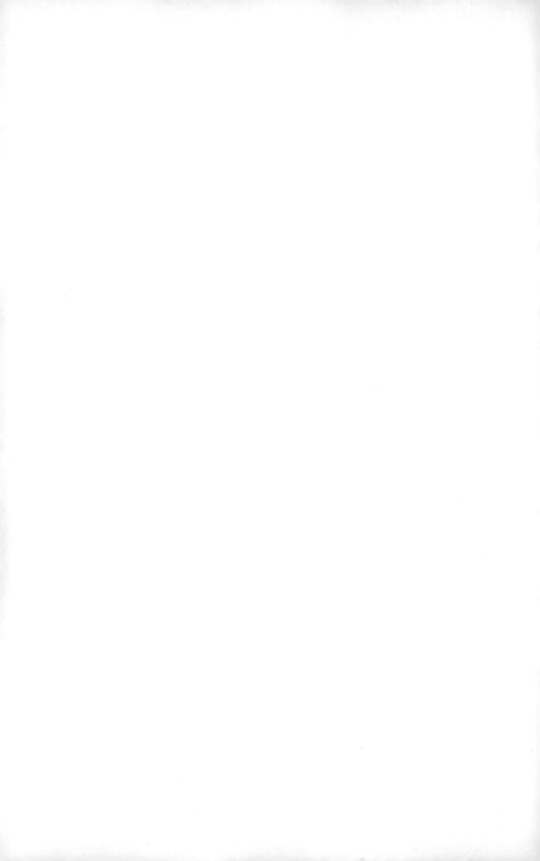

*Chapter 8*

# ULTRASOUND

## Contact Technique

### *I. Preparations*

A. Determine the procedure to be used:
    1. Contact technique:
        a. This technique is used on relatively smooth muscular surfaces and where some light but complete

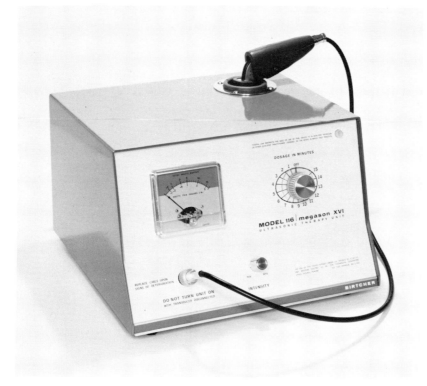

Figure 17. Megason ultrasound. (Courtesy of the Birtcher Corp.)

transducer pressure can be tolerated.
  b. The transducer remains in contact with the skin throughout the treatment.
  c. A coupling medium must be used between the skin and transducer.
2. Moving transducer:
  a. The transducer is kept moving on the skin throughout the treatment.
  b. Continuous or pulsed ultrasound may be used.
3. Stationary transducer:
  a. The transducer is put on the skin and left in place throughout the treatment.
  b. Pulsed ultrasound *must* be used with a 13 cm² or smaller transducer.
B. Check the unit to be used:
  1. The unit must be grounded.
  2. Know how to operate the unit.
  3. All switches should be off.
  4. Transducer and plug connections should be tight.
  5. The face of the transducer should be clean.
  6. Do *not* use a unit that is not operating properly.
  7. Make *sure* the intensity control is off, and warm up the unit if necessary.
C. Have all materials ready to use:
  1. Coupling medium:
    a. A commercially made gel is the preferred coupling medium because it will more readily adhere to the skin.
    b. A thick lotion may be used.
    c. Mineral oil is the least desirable choice. It will not adhere to the skin, and it should be removed with alcohol.

## II. Starting the Treatment

A. If the patient complains of pain during the treatment:
  1. The first thing to do is to turn the intensity to zero, add

more coupling medium, and resume treatment.
   2. If pain persists, reduce the intensity.
   3. If using the moving transducer technique, move the transducer a little faster.
   4. If these steps fail to stop the pain, terminate the treatment.
B. *Never* treat *any* part of *any* patient who has an external or implanted atomic or electrical device of any kind. The high frequency current in the transducer cable that causes the transducer crystal to vibrate may alter the operation of the device.
C. Explain the procedure to the patient:
   1. Tell him how long the treatment will be.
   2. Tell him he may not feel anything.
   3. Emphasize that he should tell you *immediately* if he has *any* pain or burning in the area being treated.
   4. Show the patient the coupling medium you will use.
D. Check the area to be treated:
   1. The skin should be clean, dry, and free from oils, lotions, creams, etc.
   2. Check skin sensation. If sensation is diminished or lacking, use low intensity.
   3. Avoid treating on abrasions, recent scar tissue, new skin, etc.
   4. Do *not* treat on bony prominences.
   5. Do *not* treat over or near the heart.
   6. If treating a large area, divide it into sections and treat each section separately:
      a. When using a 13 cm² or smaller transducer, the treatment area should be no more than 6 by 6 inches. The smaller the transducer surface, the smaller the area should be.
      b. When using a 50 cm² *moving* transducer, the treatment area may be 12 by 12 inches.
      c. When using a 50 cm² *stationary* transducer, the treatment area must be the same size as the transducer.

E.  Tell the patient you are going to put some gel (lotion) onto his skin and that it will feel cold.

F.  Apply *room temperature* or cooler coupling medium *liberally* and directly onto the skin:

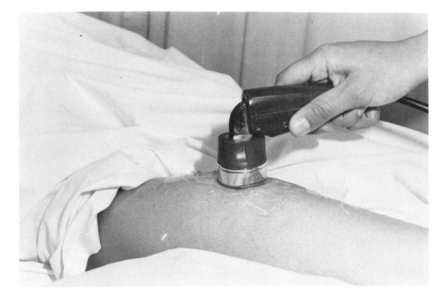

Figure 18. Contact technique using a gel.

1.  Protect any remaining clothing the patient has on from the coupling medium.
2.  Be sure the patient is not sensitive to the coupling medium. This may not be discovered until after the first treatment.
3.  *Never* warm up the coupling medium. When the coupling medium is cool, more heat is lost through the skin.
4.  Too much coupling medium is better than too little.
5.  Warn the patient and using transducer, spread the coupling medium over the skin.
6.  It is essential that the face of the transducer be completely covered with the coupling medium.
7.  Do *not* place the coupling medium container on top of the unit.

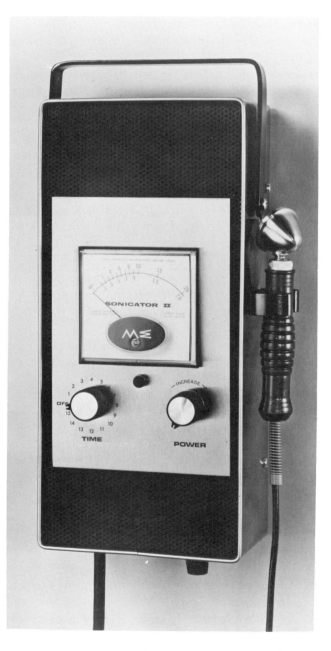

Figure 19. Sonicator II ultrasound. (Courtesy of Mettler Electronics Corp.)

G. Recheck to be sure the intensity control is off.
H. Turn on the unit (unless preheated).
I. Set the unit automatic timer to the desired treatment time. Treatment time is usually five minutes.
J. To increase the intensity when the transducer is moving:
    1. Recheck to be sure there is enough coupling medium on the skin and transducer.
    2. Apply the transducer to the skin:
        a. Transducer pressure should be complete but *not* heavy. Pressure caused by the weight of the regular transducer is sufficient.
        b. Complete contact is essential.
        c. The transducer *must* be held at a *right angle* to the skin being treated, and the right angle must be maintained *throughout* the treatment.
    3. With the transducer *constantly moving* in any direction and in firm contact with the skin, quickly adjust the intensity control to the desired watts per centimeter squared (or total watts as indicated by the manufacturer of the unit you are using):
        a. The 13 cm² or smaller transducer *cannot* remain stationary while adjusting the intensity. (With some units, the intensity may be set while the transducer is in its holder.)
        b. If the treatment is for five minutes, the intensity is usually 1 w/cm² or less.
        c. Be *sure* to read the correct meter scale. The *lower* scale is usually w/cm².
K. Treatment using a moving transducer:
    1. If you have used your dominant hand to adjust the intensity control, quickly transfer the transducer to that hand.
    2. Constantly move the transducer in either small circles or short longitudinal strokes:
        a. The speed of the movement is *slow* — about 1 inch per second.
        b. The next stroke should cover 50 percent of the previous stroke. Do *not* stroke forward and then back in

the same place or make a second circle in the same place as the first circle.

L. To increase the intensity when the transducer is stationary:
1. Pulsed ultrasound *must* be used with transducers less than 13 cm² in size.
2. A gel coupling medium *must* be used with any size transducer.
3. Position the transducer on the skin:
   a. Excellent contact is essential.
   b. The transducer should be at a *right angle* to the skin.
4. Increase the intensity to the desired level. Read the correct meter scale.

M. *Never* hold the transducer in the air with the intensity up from zero for more than a few seconds at any one time:
1. The face of the transducer can become hot, and the patient can be burned when the transducer is placed on the skin.
2. The transducer crystal can be damaged.
3. The glue holding the crystal to the posterior surface of the transducer face can become soft.
4. Some large transducers, 50 cm², will not become hot or damaged if the total wattage intensity is low. However, the transducer should *always* be checked for heat before continuing treatment.

N. The coupling medium *must* be kept on the skin and transducer throughout the treatment. Transducer movement will spread the coupling medium thereby enlarging the treatment area. Occasionally tip the transducer on its edge and push the coupling medium back onto the area being treated. Do *not* hold the transducer in this position for more than a few seconds at a time.

### III. Terminating the Treatment

A. The unit will shut off automatically at the end of the treatment time.
B. Turn the intensity control back to zero. If treatment must

be discontinued before the unit shuts off, keep the transducer moving on the skin while turning the intensity to
zero.

C.  Wipe off the coupling medium from the transducer and
replace it in its holder, making sure it is secure.

D.  Move the unit to the back of the treatment booth out of the
patient's way.

E.  Wipe off the coupling medium from the skin. If mineral oil
has been used, put some alcohol on a towel and take off the
oil.

F.  Thoroughly check the patient's skin.

### UNDERWATER TECHNIQUE

### *I. Preparations*

A.  Determine the procedure to be used:
   1. Underwater technique:
      a. This technique is used when the surface is uneven

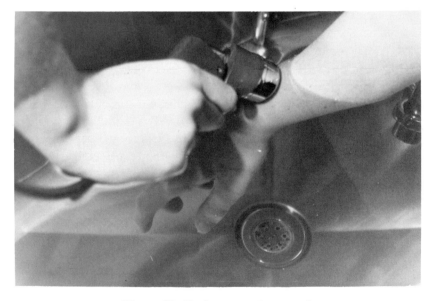

Figure 20. Underwater ultrasound.

such as the hand, elbow, knee, ankle, etc., where good contact between the transducer and skin is not possible or where the area to be treated is sensitive to pressure such as amputation stumps.
   b. The part to be treated and the transducer are immersed in water.
   c. The coupling medium is the water.
   d. The transducer is held from 1/2 to 1 inch from the skin.
  2. Select continuous or pulsed ultrasound.
  3. Moving transducer:
   a. The transducer is kept moving on the skin throughout the treatment.
   b. Continuous or pulsed ultrasound may be used.
  4. Stationary transducer:
   a. The transducer is put 1/2 to 1 inch from the skin and left in place throughout the treatment. This technique is very difficult to use under water.
   b. Pulsed ultrasound must be used with the 13 cm$^2$ or smaller transducers.
   c. Continuous or pulsed ultrasound may be used with the 50 cm$^2$ transducers.
B.  Check the unit to be used:
  1. The unit must be grounded.
  2. Know how to operate the unit.
  3. All switches should be off.
  4. Transducer and plug connections should be tight.
  5. The transducer *must* be waterproof.
  6. The face of the transducer should be clean.
  7. Do not use a unit that is not operating properly.
  8. Make sure the intensity control is off, and warm up the unit if necessary.
C.  Have all materials ready to use:
  1. A container will be needed that is large enough to immerse the part to be treated, the transducer and the therapist's hand.
  2. A whirlpool may be used:
   a. The turbine should be plugged in, grounded and

*off.*
b. No part of the turbine or whirlpool tank should come in contact with the ultrasound unit.
c. Do not allow the patient to touch the ultrasound unit while he is being treated.

3. The water temperature should be no more than 70° F.

## II. Starting the Treatment

A. Be sure the patient does not touch any metal such as a sink, electrical outlet, etc.
B. If the patient complains of pain during the treatment:
   1. The first thing to do is to reduce the intensity.
   2. If pain persists and if the moving transducer technique is being used, move the transducer a little faster.
   3. If these steps fail to stop the pain, terminate treatment.
D. *Never* treat *any* part of *any* patient who has an external or implanted atomic or electrical device of any kind. The high frequency current in the transducer cable that causes the transducer crystal to vibrate may alter the operation of the device.
D. Explain the procedure to the patient:
   1. Tell him how long the treatment will be.
   2. Tell him he may not feel anything although ultra-sound is felt more readily in water. If he does not feel anything and you want to assure him he is getting something:
      a. Reduce the intensity to zero.
      b. Be sure no part of the patient is in the water.
      c. Hold the transducer 1 inch under the water with the face pointed toward the surface.
      d. Increase the intensity until ripples can be seen.
      e. If the transducer face is barely under the water and the intensity is high, fog or mist will appear.
      f. This same technique may be used if the patient does not feel anything with the contact technique.
   3. Explain to him that he should tell you *immediately* if he has *any* pain or burning in the treatment area.

E. Check the area to be treated:
   1. The skin should be clean, dry, and free from lotions, creams, oils, etc.
   2. Check skin sensation. If sensation is lacking or diminished, use lower intensity than normal.
   3. Avoid treating on abrasions, recent scar tissue or new skin.
   4. Do *not* treat on bony prominences.
   5. Do *not* treat over or near the heart.
   6. If treating a large area, divide it into sections and treat each area separately:
      a. When using a 13 cm$^2$ or smaller transducer, the treatment area should be no more than 6 by 6 inches.
F. Have (help) the patient immerse the part in the water:
   1. The water must completely surround the area to be treated.
   2. Remind the patient not to move as this can create air bubbles.
   3. Allow the patient to remain in the water without moving for a few minutes before starting treatment to allow all of the air bubbles to dissipate.
G. Slowly immerse the transducer into the water:
   1. The face of the transducer must be completely covered with the water throughout the treatment.
   2. *Never* touch the skin with the transducer when the intensity is up from zero.
   3. Be sure there are no air bubbles on the skin or the face of the transducer. Putting alcohol on the skin and face of the transducer before putting them into the water will help reduce the accumulation of air bubbles.
H. Recheck to be sure the intensity control is at zero.
I. Select continuous or pulsed ultrasound (unless done).
J. Turn on the unit (unless preheated).
K. Set the unit automatic timer to the desired treatment time.
L. The 13 cm$^2$ or smaller transducer *cannot* remain stationary while the intensity is adjusted (With some units, the intensity may be set while the transducer is in its holder.):
   1. With the transducer *constantly moving,* quickly adjust

the intensity control to the desired watts per square centimeter (or total watts) as indicated by the manufacturer of the unit you are using:

    a. If the treatment is for five minutes, the intensity is usually 1 w/cm² or less.

    b. Be *sure* to read the *correct* meter scale. The lower scale is usually w/cm², and the upper scale is total watts.

M. Treatment using a moving transducer:

    1. If you have used your dominant hand to adjust the intensity, quickly transfer the transducer to that hand.

    2. Constantly move the transducer back and forth parallel to the part in small longitudinal strokes. These movements are easier to control under water than are circular strokes:

        a. The speed of the movement is *slow* — about 1 inch per second.

        b. The next stroke should cover only 50 percent of the previous stroke. Do *not* stroke forward and then back in the same place.

N. Care must be taken when the transducer is under water in a metal tank with the intensity up from zero as the ultrasound is reflected by the metal.

O. *Never* take the transducer out of the water with the intensity up from zero for more than a few seconds at any one time:

    1. Air will reflect the ultrasound back to the face of the transducer making it hot.

    2. The transducer crystal can be damaged.

    3. The glue holding the crystal to the posterior surface of the transducer face can become soft.

    4. Some large transducers, 50 cm², will not become hot or damaged if the total wattage intensity is low. However the transducer should *always* be checked for heat before continuing treatment.

P. When air bubbles appear on the skin and/or transducer face, they should be wiped away *immediately* with your hand.

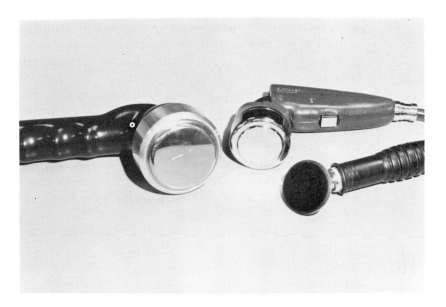

Figure 21. Ultrasound transducers.

### III. Terminating the Treatment

A. The unit will shut off automatically at the end of the treatment time.

B. Turn the intensity control back to zero. If treatment must be discontinued before the unit's automatic timer activates the off switch, keep the transducer moving until the intensity is at zero.

C. Dry the transducer thoroughly and return it to its holder.

D. Move the unit back out of the patient's way.

E. Have (help) the patient thoroughly dry his skin.

F. Check the patient's skin.

## COUPLING CUSHION TECHNIQUE

### I. Preparations

A. Determine the procedure to be used:

1. Coupling cushion technique:
   a. This technique is used to treat irregular surfaces that cannot be submerged in water such as the shoulder.
   b. A thin rubber or plastic bag may be used as the cushion.
   c. A gel coupling medium *must* be used between the cushion and the skin and between the cushion and the transducer.
   d. The transducer remains in contact with the cushion throughout the treatment.
2. Moving transducer:
   a. The transducer is constantly in motion on the cushion.
   b. Continuous or pulsed ultrasound may be used regardless of the size of the transducer.
3. Stationary transducers:
   a. The transducer is put on the cushion and left in place throughout the treatment. This technique is very difficult to use with the coupling cushion.
   b. Pulsed ultrasound *must* be used with a 13 cm² or smaller transducer.
B. Check the unit to be used:
   1. The unit must be grounded.
   2. Know how to operate the unit.
   3. All switches should be off.
   4. Transducer and plug connections should be tight.
   5. The face of the transducer should be clean.
   6. Do *not* use a unit that is not operating properly.
   7. Make *sure* the intensity control is off, and warm up the unit if necessary.
C. Prepare the coupling cushion:
   1. Ideally, the water used to fill the cushion should be boiled to remove the air, and then allowed to cool.
   2. It is usually not possible to boil the water, so fill a container such as a plastic dishpan with cold water.
   3. Allow the water to stand for about twenty minutes or until the air bubbles have dissipated.
   4. Roll up the cushion to remove all of the air.

5. Slowly immerse the rolled up cushion in the water.
6. Keeping the cushion under the water, slowly unroll it and allow it to fill.
7. When the cushion has filled and keeping it under the water, put an elastic band around the open end of the cushion and tighten it slightly.
8. While the cushion is still underwater, squeeze it gently to allow some water to escape. The cushion should be about 80 percent full of water.
9. Still under water, tighten the elastic band to completely close the opening.

D. Have all towels, etc. ready to use.

## II. *Starting the Treatment*

A. If the patient complains of pain during the treatment:
   1. The first thing to do is to reduce the intensity. Then add more coupling medium between the cushion and skin, and cushion and transducer.
   2. If pain persists and the moving transducer is being used, move the transducer a little faster.
   3. If these procedures fail to stop the pain, terminate the treatment.
B. *Never* treat *any* part of *any* patient who has an external or implanted atomic or electrical device of any kind. The high frequency current in the transducer cable that causes the crystal to vibrate may alter the operation of the device.
C. Explain the procedure to the patient:
   1. Tell him how long the treatment will be.
   2. Tell him that he may not feel anything.
   3. Explain to him that he should tell you *immediately* if he has *any* pain or burning sensation in the area being treated.
   4. Show the patient the gel you will use.
D. Check the area to be treated:
   1. The skin should be clean, dry, and free from lotions, oils, creams, etc.
   2. Check skin sensation. If sensation is lacking or dimin-

ished, use lower intensity than normal.
3. Avoid treating on abrasions, recent scar tissue or new skin.
4. Do *not* treat bony prominences.
5. Do *not* treat over or near the heart.
6. The treatment area will be the same size as the cushion.

E.  Tell the patient you are going to put the gel onto his skin and that it will feel cool.

F.  Apply *room temperature* gel *liberally* and directly onto his skin:
1. *Never* warm up the coupling medium.
2. Be sure the patient is not sensitive to the gel. You may not discover this until after the first treatment.
3. Protect any remaining clothing from the gel.
4. Too much gel is better than too little.
5. Warn the patient and using the transducer, spread the gel over the skin.

G.  Apply the gel *liberally* to the side of the cushion that will touch the patient. Spread the gel over the cushion with the transducer.

H.  Place the cushion on the area to be treated.

I.  Hold the cushion in place with one hand, and apply the gel to the top side of the cushion. With the transducer, spread the gel evenly over the cushion.

J.  Check to be sure the transducer face is completely covered with the gel.

K.  Recheck to be sure the intensity control is off.

L.  Turn on the unit (unless preheated).

M.  Set the unit timer for the desired treatment time. Treatment time is usually five minutes.

N.  Place the transducer on the cushion:
1. Transducer contact must be light but complete.
2. Hold and maintain the transducer at a *right angle*.

O.  With the transducer moving in small, circular movements, adjust the intensity to the desired watts per square centimeter or total watts:
1. Assistance may be required. Do not allow the cushion to slip.

2. The intensity is usually 1 w/cm² or less.
3. Read the *correct* meter scale.
4. Each circular movement should cover one half of the previous circle.

P.  *Never* hold the transducer in the air with the intensity up from zero:

    1. The face of the transducer can become hot, and the patient can be burned when the transducer is placed on the skin.

    2. The transducer crystal can be damaged.

    3. The glue holding the crystal to the posterior surface of the transducer face can become soft.

    4. Some large transducers, 50 cm², will not become hot or damaged if the total wattage intensity is low. However, the transducer should *always* be checked for heat before continuing treatment.

Q.  The coupling medium *must* be kept on the skin, transducer and cushion throughout the treatment. Occasionally, tip the transducer on its edge and push the gel back onto the center of the bag.

### III. Terminating the Treatment

A.  The unit will shut off automatically at the end of the treatment time set.

B.  Turn the intensity control back to zero. If treatment must be discontinued before the unit shuts off, keep the transducer moving while turning the intensity to zero.

C.  Wipe off the gel from the transducer, the cushion and from the patient's skin.

D.  Move the unit back out of the patient's way.

E.  Check the patient's skin.

F.  Empty the water from the bag.

G.  Wash the bag in lukewarm water using a mild soap.

## Chapter 9

# SHORT WAVE DIATHERMY

## *I. Preparations*

A. Determine the procedure to be used:
    1. Induction (electromagnetic) field heating:
        a. Drum.
        b. Cable.
        c. Flexible inductance electrode.
    2. Condenser (electric) field heating:
        a. Air-spaced/condenser plates.
        b. Condenser pads.
        c. Condenser cuffs.
B. Check the unit to be used:
    1. The unit must be grounded.
    2. Know how to operate the unit and electrodes.
    3. All dials should be off.
    4. All adjustments, manual or automatic, should be in working order.
    5. Do *not* use frayed line cords or electrode cables, electrodes or improperly functioning equipment.
    6. All plug and electrode connections must be tight.
    7. Warm up the unit if necessary.
    8. Make sure the unit is operating safely and efficiently.
C. Have all necessary materials ready to use:
    1. Proper electrodes.
    2. Linen.

## *II. Starting the Treatment*

A. Explain the procedure to the patient:
    1. Tell him how long the treatment will be.
    2. Explain that the sensation he *should* feel should be one of warmth and *not* heat. It should be a velvety, smooth

warmth and not a burning sensation.

    3. He should call you *immediately* if he becomes uncomfortable because of improper support, pain, burning, too hot, etc.

    4. He should not move until the unit has been turned off.

B. *Never treat any part of any patient who has an external or implanted atomic or electrical device of any kind.*

C. Check the skin on the area to be treated:

    1. The skin should be clean, dry, and free from oils, lotions, creams, etc.

    2. If there are any unusual marks, do not treat until you know what they are.

    3. Do not treat on new skin, recent scar tissue, etc.

D. Check skin sensation. If sensation is lacking or diminished, use short wave with *extreme* caution or not at all.

E. *There can be no metal in or near the treatment field*:

    1. *Never* treat a patient on a metal bed or one with metal springs, or in a metal chair. Metal chair seats, arms, and/or legs are absolute contraindications for using short wave.

    2. *Never* use short wave over or near a metal implant such as metal plate, intrauterine device, metal sutures, etc.

    3. External hearing aides should be removed and placed at least 4 feet from the treatment field.

    4. Jewelry, belt buckles, bobby pins in hair or wigs, bra clips, zippers, safety pins, etc. *must* be removed from the treatment field.

    5. Do *not* treat near or on the face of a patient with metal braces on his face. However, metal fillings in the teeth are not contraindications for treating the face.

    6. Any unremovable metal that will be in the treatment field, such as a wedding ring, is an absolute contraindication for using short wave.

    7. Some therapists advocate never using short wave on any part of a patient who has metal in him anywhere in his body.

F. If treating the hand, wrist or forearm or if the wrist will be near the treatment field, the patient's watch should be removed (nonmagnetic or not). The therapist should remove his watch unless it is nonmagnetic.

G. Contact lenses should be removed when treating the face.

H. *There can be no moisture in the area:*

1. The skin on the area to be treated *must* be dry and free from perspiration.

2. Two different skin surfaces should be separated with six layers of heavy turkish toweling or treated separately. Examples: (1) If treating the shoulder, pad the axilla with toweling; (2) If treating both knees at the same time, place six layers of turkish toweling between them or wrap each knee separately.

3. *Never* use wet or damp toweling, sheets, etc.

I. Do *not* use short wave unless you can see the skin. Bandages, casts, splints, dressings, etc. are contraindications for short wave.

J. *Never* use two short wave diathermy units on the same patient at the same time.

K. *Never* use short wave on a patient at the same time you are using another modality, for safety reasons. Use each separately.

L. Do *not* use short wave over the pelvic area during menstruation or pregnancy.

M. Warn the patient about touching the unit, the electrode, any metal, the conducting cord or any electrical outlet.

## Induction or Electromagnetic Field Heating

N. Drum (curved, hinged, molded, or round):

1. Place one layer of turkish toweling on the area to be treated for hygienic purposes and to absorb perspiration.

2. Make sure the drum cables are unplugged from the unit.

3. Position the drum over the toweling:

a. Raise or lower the retaining arm as necessary.

b. Leave approximately 1/2 inch of space between the drum and towel. Some manufacturers recommend

that the drum be placed in contact with the patient.
   c. Extra padding may be required over bony promi-
      nences and under the drum corners and edges.
   d. The closer the drum is to the skin, the less will be
      the intensity needed.
4. Plug in the electrode cables:
   a. Be sure to select the correct receptacles.
   b. The drum cables should go between the drum arm
      and the patient.
   c. Whether they touch or not, the cables must *not* cross
      each other.
5. The cables cannot come in contact with each other (on
   older units), the drum, the patient, any part of the unit
   or the plinth pad:
   a. Use the cable retainers on the drum arm.
   b. Use six layers of turkish toweling to pad the cables.
O. Cable wrap around (used around the extremities):
   1. Use six layers of turkish toweling for padding:
      a. Unfold three large turkish towels, and put one on
         top of the other.

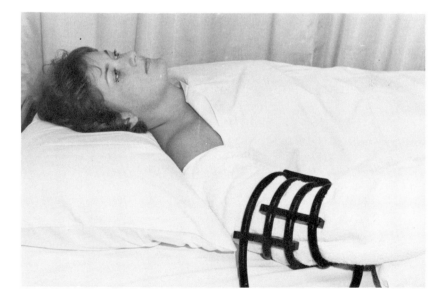

Figure 22. Cable wrap around.

    b. Wrap the extremity (knee, ankle, elbow) in the three towels. All skin surfaces on the area to be treated *must* be padded with at least six layers of toweling.

2. Form the cable into at least three loops, and slide it over the extremity, or the cable may be wrapped around the extremity one loop at a time.
3. The cable ends should be even in length.
4. The cable loops should fit snuggly but should not be tight.
5. Each loop must be kept at least 1 inch from another loop:
   a. Use spacers if available. Avoid putting spacers under the extremity.
   b. Padding should be used between the loops if spacers are not available. The padding must be thick and securely anchored to prevent any possible contact of the loops.
6. The cable ends should be padded with at least six layers of turkish toweling to prevent possible contact with each other, the patient, any part of the unit or the plinth pad.
7. Plug the cables into the correct unit receptacles.

P. Pancake coil (used principally on the back):
1. Form the cable into a flat coil corresponding to the size of the area to be treated.
2. The coil should have at least three circles.
3. The ends of the coil should be even in length.
4. No part of the cable may touch another part, the patient, the unit or the plinth pad:
   a. Separate the coils with spacers. Use at least three spacers, and distribute them evenly around the coil.
   b. Place the rubber insulation sleeve around the cable leading from the center of the circle. If the sleeve is not available, use six layers of turkish toweling. This part of the cable must *not* come in contact with the coils.
5. Place six layers of turkish toweling on the area to be

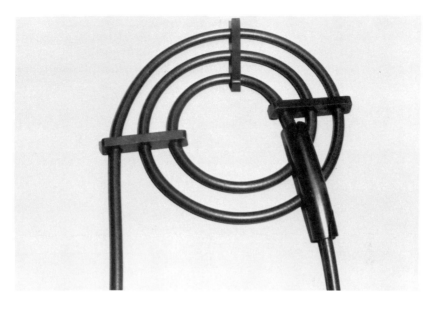

Figure 23. Pancake coil.

    treated.
6. Place the coil on the toweling.
7. Hold the coil in place with a light sandbag.
8. Plug the cables into the correct receptacles.
9. Use at least six layers of turkish toweling to pad the ends of the cable to prevent possible contact with each other, the patient, the unit, or the plinth pad.
Q. Flexible inductance electrode (used principally on the back):
    1. Place six layers of turkish toweling on the area to be treated.
    2. Place the electrode on the toweling.
    3. Hold the electrode in place with a light sandbag.
    4. Use at least six layers of turkish toweling to keep the electrode cables at least 5 inches apart and to prevent contact with each other, the patient, the unit, or plinth pad.
    5. Plug the cables into the currect unit receptacles.

## Electric or Condenser Field Heating

R. Air-spaced or condenser plates:
   1. Both plates must be used at the same time.
   2. The two plates are mounted on adjustable arms and can be retained in any position.

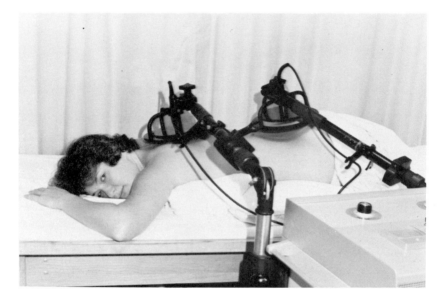

Figure 24. Air spaced plates. (Burkick Corp. unit)

   3. The distance between the plate and the guard are adjustable. The spacing between the plate and the patient is usually 1 inch.
   4. Adjust the plates over the area to be treated:
      a. Use the adjustment knobs, and raise or lower the retaining arms as necessary.
      b. The plates should be parallel to the skin.
      c. Usually, toweling is not used between the plates and the skin. If perspiration appears, immediately reduce the intensity to zero and wipe off the moisture.
      d. The plates may be placed side by side on the same

surface providing they can be kept at least 10 inches apart, or one plate may be placed on the anterior surface of the area to be treated and the other plate on the posterior surface (medial and lateral).

5. Plug the plate cables into the correct unit receptacles:
    a. The cables *cannot* come in contact with each other, the electrode arms, the patient or any part of the unit or plinth pad. Use six layers of turkish toweling and/or the cable retainers.
    b. The cables cannot cross each other.

S. Condenser pads:
    1. Both pads must be used at the same time.
    2. Place six layers of turkish toweling on the area to be treated.

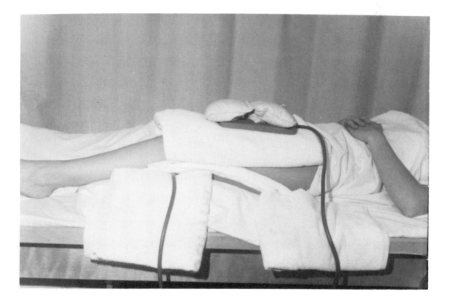

Figure 25. Condenser pads.

3. Place the pads on the toweling:
    a. The pads may be placed side by side on the same surface, and they should be kept as far apart as pos-

sible.

    b. One pad may be placed on the anterior surface and the other on the posterior surface (medial and lateral).

    c. *Never* place the pads under the patient if treating the trunk. One pad may be placed under an extremity, but more padding will be necessary.

    d. Light sandbags may be used to hold the pads in place.

T. Condenser cuffs (used on extremities):

    1. Both cuffs must be used at the same time.

    2. Wrap six layers of turkish toweling around the part.

    3. Wrap the cuffs around the toweling:

        a. Overlapping the ends of the cuffs makes no difference.

        b. The cuffs should be at least 5 inches apart.

    4. Hold the cuffs in place with rubber straps or an Ace® bandage. Metal fasteners or pins should not be used to secure the straps or bandage.

    5. Plug the cuff cables into the correct unit receptacles.

U. Turn on the unit if it has not been preheated.

V. Push the reset switch (if there is one).

W. Recheck to be sure that all insulation is in place and that the patient is relaxed and comfortable.

X. Ask the patient to tell you when he *begins* to feel a velvety, warm sensation, and increase the intensity to the lowest level of the treatment area on the unit meter:

    1. Tune the unit (if necessary).

    2. The patient will not necessarily feel warmth until the unit is tuned (manual tuning) and/or the intensity has been increased.

    3. To tune a unit, *slowly* turn the tuning dial back and forth clockwise and counterclockwise until the meter indicator reaches its highest excursion. Leave it at this point.

    4. If the patient does not feel warmth and the intensity is in the safe range as indicated by the meter, do *not*

increase the intensity. Remember that the meter is no indicator of how much current the patient is getting.

    5. If the patient feels warmth when the meter indicator is in the lower limits of the safe range for that unit, leave the intensity at that point.

Y. If the intensity is reduced to zero for any reason, the unit should *always* be retuned when continuing treatment if necessary for that unit. *Always* turn the intensity to zero when adjusting or moving the electrodes for *any* reason, because you can be burned.

Z. Treatment time is usually twenty to thirty minutes.

## III. Terminating the Treatment

A. Turn the intensity control to zero.

B. Turn the tuning control to off.

C. Turn off the main switch. Some units will be shut off automatically by the timer. If this occurs, remember to turn all controls to zero and push the reset switch. In case of overload, some units will shut off automatically, and the reset switch will have to be activated before the unit will operate.

D. Remove the electrodes and padding.

E. Move the unit to the back of the booth out of the patient's way. Do not move the unit by holding onto the electrodes.

F. Thoroughly check the patient's skin.

### AUTO*THERM®

### Mettler Electronics Corporation

## I. Preparations

A. Determine the procedure to be used.

B. Check the unit:

    1. The unit must be grounded.

    2. Know how to operate the unit.

3. All dials should be off.

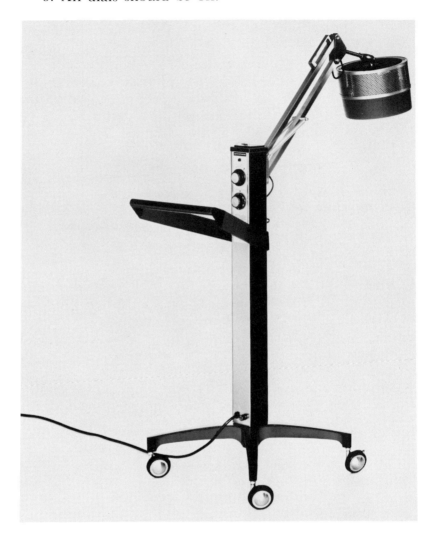

Figure 26. Auto*Therm. (Courtesy of Mettler Electronics Corp.)

4. Do *not* use a frayed line cord, defective electrode or an improperly functioning unit.
5. All adjustments, manual or automatic, should be in

working order.
6. All connections should be tight.
7. Make sure the unit is operating safely and efficiently.

## II. *Starting the Treatment*

A. *Never* treat *any* part of *any* patient who has an external or implanted atomic or electrical stimulating device of any kind.
B. Explain the procedure to the patient:
1. Tell him how long the treatment will be.
2. The sensation he *should* feel should be one of velvety warmth and *not* heat.
3. He should call you *immediately* if he becomes uncomfortable because of improper support, the treatment is too hot, pain, etc.
4. He should not move until the unit has been turned off.
C. Check the skin on the area to be treated:
1. The skin should be clean, dry, and free from lotions, oils, creams, etc.
2. If there are any unusual marks, do not treat until you know what they are.
3. Do not treat on new skin, recent scar tissue, etc.
D. Check skin sensation. If sensation is lacking or diminished, use short wave with *extreme* caution or not at all.
E. *There can be no metal in or near the treatment field*:
1. *Never* treat a patient on a metal bed or one with metal springs or in a metal chair. Metal chair seats, arms and/or legs are absolute contraindications for short wave.
2. *Never* use the Auto*Therm over or near a metal implant such as a metal plate, intrauterine device, metal sutures, etc.
3. Belt buckles, jewelry, bobby pins in hair or wigs, bra clips, zippers, safety pins, etc. must be removed from the treatment field.
4. Do *not* treat on or near the face of a patient with metal

braces on his teeth. However, metal fillings in the teeth are not contraindications for treating the face.

   5. Any unremovable metal that will be in the treatment field, such as a wedding ring, is a contraindication for treatment with short wave.
   6. Some therapists advocate never using short wave on any part of a patient who has metal in him anywhere.

F.  If treating the hand, wrist, or forearm or if the wrist will be near the treatment field, the patient's watch should be removed (nonmagnetic or not). The therapist should remove his watch unless it is nonmagnetic.

G.  Contact lenses should be removed when treating the face.

H.  *There can be no moisture in the area:*
   1. The skin on the area to be treated *must* be dry and free from perspiration.
   2. Two different skin surfaces should be separated with six layers of heavy turkish toweling or treated separately. Examples: (1) If treating the shoulder, pad the axilla with toweling; (2) If treating both knees at the same time, place six layers of turkish toweling between them.
   3. *Never* use damp or wet toweling, sheets, etc.

I.  Do *not* use the Auto*Therm unless you can easily see the bare skin. Bandages, casts, splints, dressings, etc. are contraindications for short wave.

J.  *Never* use two short wave diathermy units on the same patient at the same time.

K.  *Never* use short wave on a patient at the same time you are using another modality. Use each modality by itself.

L.  Do *not* use the Auto*Therm over the pelvic area during menstruation or pregnancy.

M.  Warn the patient about touching the unit, the electrode, any metal, the conducting cord or any electrical outlets.

N.  Place a single layer of turkish toweling on the skin to be treated for hygienic purposes and to absorb perspiration.

O.  Position the treatment drum *on* the toweling. Extra padding may be required over bony prominences and under the drum edge.

P. Set the unit timer to the desired treatment time:
   1. The timer activates the unit.
   2. Some units require a thirty second warm-up time.
Q. Increase the intensity to the manufacturer's recommended wattage for the area being treated and/or to the patient's tolerance:
   1. Manufacturer's recommended wattage: ankle — 9; cervical — 21; chest — 24; ear — 9; eye and sinus — 9; elbow — 13; feet — 11 to both, 6 to each; forearm — 10; hand — 5; hip — 23; knee — 18; pelvis — 26; lumbar area — 28; shoulder — 23.
R. The unit is tuned automatically.
S. *Always* turn the intensity to zero when adjusting or removing the drum before the unit is shut off by the timer.
T. Treatment time is usually twenty to thirty minutes.

### III. *Terminating the Treatment*

A. The automatic timer will shut off the unit.
B. Turn the intensity control to zero.
C. Remove the drum.
D. Move the unit to the back of the treatment booth out of the patient's way.
E. Check the patient's skin.

### IV. *Notes*

A. *Never* cover the ventilation holes in the treatment head.
B. *Always* replace the fuse with one of the *same* amperage.
C. Occasionally, wash the drum face with a mild soap.

## Chapter 10

# MICROWAVE

## *I. Preparations*

A. Determine the procedure to be used:
    1. Select the directors:
        a. Directors should be selected for the shape and size of the heating pattern they present.

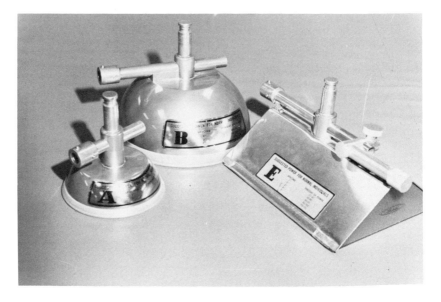

Figure 27. Microwave directors. (Burkick Corp. unit)

        b. Directors A and B are circular, and 4 and 6 inches in diameter respectively. These present a circular heating pattern with 100 percent of power being emitted halfway between the center and edge of each director. These should be used over convex and/or irregular surfaces.

c. Directors C, D, and E are rectangular. (Director D is seldom used.) These present an oval heating pattern with 100 percent of power being emitted from the center of each director. These should be used over concave and/or smooth surfaces.

2. Install the correct director:
   a. Loosen all arm adjustments before moving the arm.
   b. The arm and cable should come off the back of the unit instead of going over the control panel. It will then be easier to position the director over the patient, and there will be no danger of damaging the director because of reflection of radiation from the top of the unit.
   c. Position the end of the arm over the plinth before installing the director. Then the director will fall onto the plinth if it is dropped or not properly attached.
   d. Older units should not only be off, but they should be unplugged. On new units, the main switch should be off.
   e. Holding the director by its top, attach it to the holder on the arm. Do *not* touch the protective covering over the antennae.
   f. Attach the coaxial cable to the director.
   g. Check to make sure both connections secure.

B. *Never* use any director without its protective coverings as contact with the antenna tips can cause burns.

C. *Never* point the director at any metal with the intensity up from zero because reflection of the electromagnetic radiation from the metal into the director can damage the director.

D. Install the spacer. If the spacer is missing, have a tape measure ready to use. *Never* estimate the spacing between the skin and the director.

E. Check the unit:
   1. The unit must be grounded.
   2. Know how to operate the unit.
   3. All dials should be off.

   4. All adjustments should be in working order.

   5. All connections should be tight.

   6. *Never* use the unit if the coaxial cable is not intact.

   7. Make sure the unit is operating safely and efficiently.

F. Warm up the unit:

   1. If you are using an older model unit, the unit will require two to three minutes to warm up. Newer models require thirty seconds or less.

   2. Be sure the unit has been "reset."

   3. Turn on the main switch. The red light (old models) or amber light (new models) will come on.

   4. At the expiration of the preheating time for older models, an amber light will glow indicating the unit is ready to use.

   5. On any model, if the main switch is turned off at any time, the unit will take the original amount of time to reheat.

G. *Never* operate the unit if the fan is not working.

H. *Never* cover the vent holes on the unit.

I. Have all materials ready to use.

## II. Starting the Treatment

A. *Never treat any part of any patient who has an external or implanted electrical or atomic stimulating device of any kind.*

B. Explain the procedure to the patient:

   1. Tell him how long the treatment will be.

   2. He should feel a warm sensation. It should be a smooth warmth compared to that of a heat lamp or hot pack.

   3. He should call you *immediately* if he becomes uncomfortable because of improper support, the treatment is too hot, pain, etc.

   4. He should not move until the intensity has been reduced to zero and the director has been raised.

C. Check the area to be treated:

   1. Any edema in the area to be treated or near it is an *absolute contraindication* for microwave.

2. The skin should be clean and *must* be free from perspiration, creams, lotions, etc.
3. Do *not* treat on new skin, recent scar tissue, etc.
4. If there are any unusual marks, do not treat until you know what they are.

D. Check skin sensation. If sensation is lacking or diminished, use microwave with *extreme* caution or not at all.

E. *There can be no metal in the treatment field:*
    1. In contrast to short wave diathermy, microwave may be given to patients on a metal bed or chair. However, *no* part of the radiation can touch the metal and the part to be treated should not rest on a metal surface (not recommended).
    2. *Never* use microwave over or near a metal implant such as a plate, intrauterine device, sutures, etc.
    3. All jewelry, belt buckles, bobby pins in hair or wigs, zippers, etc. must be removed from the treatment field.
    4. Any unremovable metal, such as a wedding ring, is an absolute contraindication for microwave to that area.

F. Watches in or near the treatment field must be removed as they can become magnetized.

G. There can be no moisture in the area:
    1. The skin *must be dry and free from perspiration.*
    2. Two different skin surfaces should be separated or padded with several thicknesses of turkish toweling to absorb perspiration.

H. Do *not* treat over or near the eyes.

I. Use *great care* when treating over bony prominences.

J. Do *not* use toweling between the director and the skin. If perspiration appears on the skin, reduce the intensity to zero, move the director and wipe off the perspiration.

K. Microwave *cannot* be used over casts, splints, dressings, etc.

L. *Never* use two microwave units on the same patient at the same time.

M. *Never* use microwave over the pelvic area during pregnancy or menstruation.

N. *Never* use microwave on a patient at the same time you are using another modality. Use each modality separately.

O. Warn the patient about touching the unit, director, line cord, any metal or electrical outlets.
P. Loosen the unit arm adjustment and position the director:
  1. Do not hold onto the director or coaxial cable.
  2. The director *must* be at a *right angle* to the skin.
  3. The director should be in the center of the area.
Q. Measure the distance from the edge of the director to the highest area to be treated:
  1. The spacer may be removed from its holder, and the distance between the director and the skin may be "sighted."
  2. The spacings that may be used for that director are listed on the director.
  3. The closer the spacing, the *smaller* will be the heating pattern and the *greater* the intensity.
  4. *Never* use a spacing that is not listed on that director.
R. After the spacing has been measured, raise the spacer to prevent contact with the patient. Be careful not to move the director.
S. The power switch should be on *reset*.

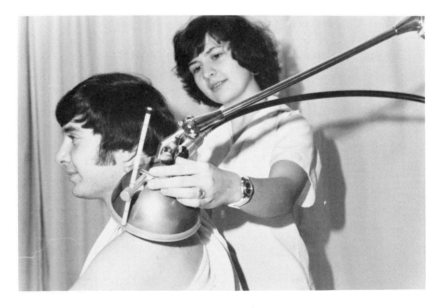

Figure 28. Microwave technique.

T. Set the unit timer:
1. On older models, a white light will glow.
2. On newer models, a red light will glow.
U. Ask the patient to tell you when he begins to feel a warm sensation.
V. Increase the intensity to the *lowest* level of the meter reading as indicated on the director for the spacing being used:
1. If the patient feels warmth *before* the meter indicates the lowest level of power, leave the intensity there.
2. If he does not feel warmth, increase the intensity within the limits indicated for the spacing you are using:
   a. Increase the intensity in steps, pausing for at least thirty seconds to allow the patient time to feel the warmth.
   b. Do *not* increase the intensity beyond the upper level of the safe range for that director at that distance.
3. If the patient feels nothing within the range of power settings for the spacing being used, reduce the intensity to zero and recheck the distance or reduce the distance if indicated for that director.

### III. Terminating the Treatment

A. The power will be shut off automatically by the timer at the end of the treatment time with the preheat switch remaining on.
B. Turn the intensity control to zero.
C. If no further treatment is to follow, turn off the main switch.
D. Loosen all arm adjustments, and move the director from over the patient.
E. Move the unit to the back of the booth out of the patient's way.
F. Thoroughly check the patient's skin.

### IV. Notes

A. The protective coverings on each director should be washed carefully with a mild soap and tepid water once a month.

# Part IV
# Cold Techniques

*Chapter 11*

# COLD WHIRLPOOL

## *I. Preparations*

A. Determine the procedure to be used
B. The room temperature should be no less than 80° F.
C. The whirlpool:
   1. Select the proper size whirlpool if available.
   2. The whirlpool must be clean.
   3. The initial water temperature depends on what part of the patient is being treated:
      a. If an upper extremity is being immersed, 55° F to 65° F temperature is usually low enough. However, it is not recommended that the temperature be lower than 50° F.
      b. If the patient is to sit in the tank, an initial temperature of no less than 80° F should be used to reduce the "shock" of immersion. Then the temperature can gradually be reduced by adding cold water to 55° or 65° F.
   4. Close the whirlpool drain.
   5. Fill the tank approximately two-thirds full of water:
      a. The turbine intakes must be well covered with water.
      b. Do not overfill. Some tanks do not have overflow drains. If the tank is too full, placing the part/patient into the water and/or turbine action will cause the water to overflow.
D. Add disinfectant if necessary:
   1. A disinfectant should be added when treating open or infected lesions.
   2. A disinfectant may be used as a psychological aid.
   3. Disposable plastic tank liners may be used. However,

special water agitation equipment may be needed.
E.  Check the turbine:
1.  The turbine must be grounded. An adapter plug with a ground wire may be used temporarily, but such an arrangement is not recommended.
2.  The line cord and plug should be in excellent condition.
3.  Be sure your hands are completely dry and that you are not standing in any water.
4.  Plug in the line cord.
5.  Be sure the air intakes on the turbine motor are not covered or clogged.
6.  Recheck the water level to be sure the turbine intakes are well covered with water.
7.  Turn on the turbine:
    a.  Adjust the water pressure and air bubbles to a soft flow.
    b.  Adjust the direction of the water flow.
8.  Turn off the turbine.
F.  Have all other materials ready to use:
1.  Whirlpool chairs and stool castors should be locked in place.
2.  Padding material and turkish towels should be ready. A turkish towel, folded several times, makes an absorbent and soft pad. Care must be taken not to allow the towel or a sponge pad to touch the water. If it does, it soon drips water onto the floor/patient.
3.  If the patient is to sit in the tank:
    a.  Appropriate clothing will be necessary.
    b.  Be sure the tank seat is secure.
    c.  Keep the patient otherwise warm.

## II. Starting the Treatment

A.  *Never* leave children, the elderly, psychotic or retarded patients unattended even for a few seconds.
B.  Be sure there is no water on the floor.
C.  Explain the procedure to the patient:

1. Show him that there is no propeller on the turbine that can hurt him.
2. Instruct him not to cover the turbine intakes on the end of the tube or those on the sides of the tube, and tell him why. (Show him these areas.)
3. Demonstrate any exercises you want him to perform while he is in the water.
4. Caution him *never* to touch any switches, the line cord, any electrical outlet or other units while he is in the water, and tell him why.

D. Have the patient remove his clothing as necessary and provide him with a T-binder, gown, bathing suit or other appropriate clothing:
1. If treating the upper extremity, have the patient remove his shirt, dress, blouse to prevent it from becoming wet from the water or perspiration. Do *not* allow the patient to roll up his sleeve as this may impair circulation.
2. If treating the leg, foot or ankle, have the patient remove his trousers or her skirt to prevent wrinkling and becoming wet. Do *not* allow the patient to roll up a pant leg.
3. When treating one leg (foot, ankle), provide a footstool or instruct the patient to put his other foot on the rungs of the whirlpool chair.
4. Provide the patient with cotton or paper scuffers to wear to and from the treatment area.

E. Have the patient remove his watch if treating the appropriate upper extremity or if the patient sits in the tank.

F. Remove all bandages, tapes, dressings, etc.:
1. These can damage an operating turbine by clogging the tube intakes.
2. Do *not* pull off dressings and bandages that stick. Allow them to soak off in the tank with the turbine off.
3. Remove them from the water before turning on the turbine.

G. Unless contraindicated, remove all braces, splints, etc. so the patient may exercise in the water.

H. Demonstrate any exercises you want the patient to perform.
I. Check skin sensation. Be sure the patient is not hypersensitive to cold.
J. Check the skin for any unusual marks, open lesions, etc.
K. Recheck the water temperature by immersing your hand in it as well as by noting the thermometer temperature.
L. Position the patient:
   1. Recheck to be sure all chair or stool castors are locked.
   2. If the patient is sitting outside of the tank, any pressure points caused by the edge of the tank should be padded.
   3. If the patient's feet will not rest comfortably on the floor, provide him with a footstool.
   4. Be sure all adjustable chairs are at the correct height.
   5. Whirlpool seat:
      a. Be sure the seat is secure. If the patient is to sit in the tank, it may be necessary to hold the seat in place until the patient steps on it or until he sits on it.
      b. If the patient's foot is being treated, he may use the seat as a footrest.
M. Position the turbine:
   1. It may be desirable to direct the water and air stream away from the part because of the diagnosis or for the first few treatments.
   2. Adjust the depth of the turbine in the water. When raising the turbine, do not pull it off its holder.
N. Be sure your hands are dry and that you are not standing in any water.
O. Turn on the turbine.
P. If patches of dead skin slough off, such as will happen when treating burns, etc., turn off the turbine several times during the treatment, remove the skin, and clean the turbine and drain strainers.
Q. Check the patient several times during the first treatment and at least once during subsequent treatments.
R. Be *sure* the patient is otherwise warm.
S. The treatment time is usually ten to twenty minutes.

### III. Terminating the Treatment

A. Turn off the turbine and move it to one side.
B. Remove the patient (extremity) from the water, and be sure he dries himself thoroughly.
C. Keep the patient warm.
D. Inspect the skin.
E. Empty and clean the tank and turbine.
F. The possibility of cross-infection must be considered:
    1. If the patient has an infected lesion, or if you have an infected or open lesion on your hands, wear rubber gloves and use a disinfectant when cleaning the tank.
    2. After removing the gloves, do *not* touch your eyes, ears, nose, or mouth until you have thoroughly washed your hands.

### IV. To sterilize a tank, see Chapter 2

*Chapter 12*

# HYDROCOLLATOR® COLD PACKS

## *I. Preparations*

A.  Determine the procedure to be used:
   1. Select the technique:
      a. Wet wrap pack. The pack is wrapped in a wet towel, which allows the patient to gradually adjust to the cold.
      b. Unwrapped pack. The wet towel is placed on the skin, and the pack is placed on the towel.
      c. Dry wrap pack. A dry towel is used between the pack and the skin.
B.  Check the unit temperature. It should be $10^0$ F.
C.  Check the packs:
   1. The packs should be cold:
      a. A thoroughly chilled pack will stay cold for approximately thirty minutes.
      b. New packs will require four to five hours to thoroughly chill.
      c. A pack that has just been returned to the unit after being used for a treatment will take at least one hour to thoroughly rechill.
   2. The proper size/shape packs should be ready to use.
   3. The pack seams should be intact.
   4. Canvas covered packs may be used with or without plastic covers.
D.  Have all other materials ready to use, such as turkish towels, water, etc.

## *II. Starting the Treatment*

A.  Explain the procedure to the patient:
   1. Tell him what the cold will feel like and why it is

120

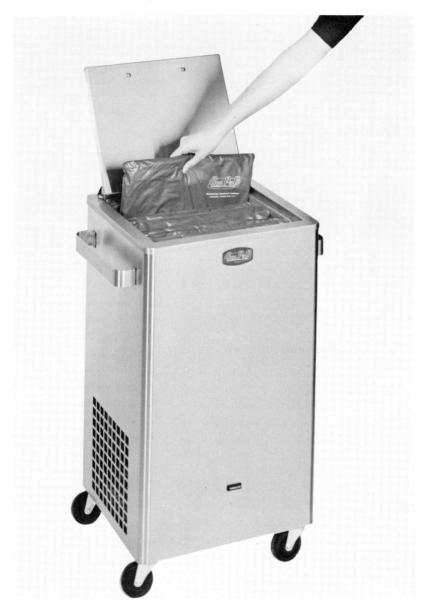

Figure 29. Col Pac chilling unit. (Courtesy of Chattanooga Pharmacal Co.)

being used.
2. Tell him he should feel only a cold sensation.
3. Explain that a towel will be placed between the pack(s) and his skin to allow him to feel the cold gradually.
4. Tell him the cold will not freeze his skin.
5. He should inform you if he has any pain or numbness or if any discomfort occurs.

B. Check the area to be treated:
1. Check skin sensation. The amount of skin sensation is usually of no concern as properly applied cold packs will not freeze the skin.
2. If the area to be treated has been frostbitten at any time, use *extreme caution* or do not use cold at all.
3. An undiagnosed rash or contagious skin disease is a contraindication for cold packs.
4. If the area to be treated is sensitive to pressure, use a small pack or use an instant cold pack.

C. Check the patient's hypersensitivity to cold. This is a *definite contraindication* to the use of cold.

D. Keep the patient otherwise warm throughout the treatment.

E. Do *not* allow the patient to lie on the pack:
1. This can become very uncomfortable and can cause pain.
2. With the use of extra pillows for the patient's comfort and support, the neck, an upper or a lower extremity may be placed on the pack unless the part is sensitive to pressure.

F. Wet wrap pack:
1. Any remaining clothing or the plinth linen should be protected from moisture.
2. If using two packs, wrap each separately. Two small packs are preferable to one large pack.
3. Dampen a turkish towel in lukewarm water. Do not use hot water, because the pack will become warm faster.
4. Wring out any excess water.
5. Spread out the towel on a flat surface.
6. Remove the correct size pack from the unit.
7. Close the unit lid.

8. Place the pack on the towel.
9. As quickly as possible, wrap the pack in the wet towel so that one side of the pack has only one layer of toweling on it.
10. Warn the patient that you are about to place the pack on his skin.
11. Gently and slowly place the pack on the skin. Do not "push" on the pack to mold it to the part.
12. Cover the pack with a dry turkish towel, and tuck it in around the part to retard warming and to hold the pack in place. Additional straps or a light sandbag may be needed to secure the pack.

G. Unwrapped pack:
1. Protect any remaining clothing and the plinth linen from moisture.

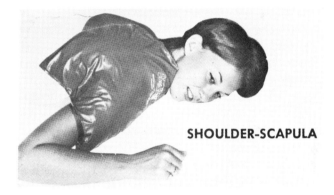

Figure 30. Cold pack. (Courtesy of Chattanooga Pharmacal Co.)

2. Two small packs are better than one large pack.
3. Dampen a turkish towel in lukewarm water. Do not use hot water because the pack will become warm faster.
4. Wring out any excess water.
5. Warn the patient that you are going to place the towel on his skin.
6. Place the towel on his skin so no more than two layers will be between the pack and the skin.

7. Remove the correct size pack from the unit.
8. Close the unit lid, and quickly place the pack on the patient.
9. Do not "push" on the pack to mold it into place.
10. Cover the pack with a dry turkish towel, and tuck it in around the patient to retard warming and to hold the pack in place. Additional straps or a light sandbag may be needed to secure the pack in place.

H. Dry wrap pack:
1. Place a dry turkish towel on a flat surface.
2. Remove the correct size pack from the unit, and place it on the towel.
3. Close the unit lid.
4. Wrap the pack so one side of the pack has only one thickness of toweling on it.
5. Warn the patient, and place the thinly wrapped side of the pack on the skin.
6. Cover the pack with a dry turkish towel, and tuck it in around the patient to retard warming and to hold the pack in place. Additional straps or a light sandbag may be needed to secure the pack.

I. No part of an unwrapped pack should touch the skin.
J. Do *not* replace the packs as they warm up. If this is necessary, the packs were not cold enough.
K. Make sure the patient is warm. Check with him frequently throughout the treatment.
L. The treatment time is usually from ten to twenty minutes.

### III. Terminating the Treatment

A. Remove the pack and toweling from the patient.
B. Give the patient a dry turkish towel and tell (help) him to dry himself thoroughly.
C. Check the patient's skin.
D. Replace the pack in the unit.

### IV. Notes

A. The unit will have to be defrosted and cleaned periodically:

1. Unplug the line cord.
2. Remove the packs.
3. Leave the unit lid open and allow the frost to melt. Do *not* chip away any ice.
4. Open the unit drain to allow melted frost to empty.
5. After the unit has defrosted, wash the insides with luke-warm water and a mild soap.
6. Rinse completely.
7. Wipe out the remaining moisture.
8. Allow the unit to dry thoroughly.
9. Replace the pack, close the unit lid and plug in the line cord.
10. Allow the packs to chill overnight.

*Chapter 13*

# INSTANT COLD PACKS

## *I. Preparations*

A.  Determine the procedure to be used:
    1. Know how to use the instant pack:
        a. Some packs are ready for use directly from the
           freezer/cold pack unit and are reusable.

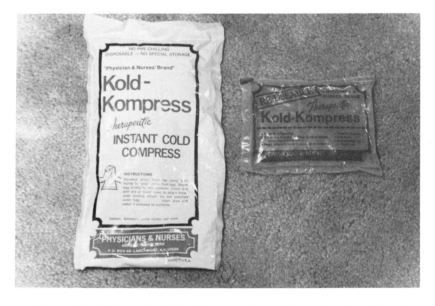

Figure 31. Cold packs. (Physicians & Nurses Manufacturing Corp.)

    b. Other instant packs are activated by breaking/
       shaking the bag(s) to mix the contents. These must
       be disposed of after using once.
    c. These packs can become expensive to use if used
       often enough (disposable packs).
    2. A light, damp handtowel should be used between any

126

pack and the skin for hygienic reasons and to allow the patient to gradually adjust to the cold.

    3. All instant packs are lightweight and easy to use.

B. Check the pack:
    1. Be sure the pack is intact.
    2. The refrigerator pack must be cold. Allow enough time between treatments for the pack to rechill.

C. Have all other materials ready to use.

## II. Starting the Treatment

A. Explain the procedure to the patient:
    1. Explain why cold is being used.
    2. Tell him he should feel only a cold sensation. Any pain or numbness should be reported to you.
    3. Explain that a towel will be used between the pack and his skin to allow him to feel the cold gradually.
    4. Tell him the cold will not freeze the skin.

B. Check the area to be treated:
    1. Skin sensation. The amount of skin sensation is usually of no concern as properly applied packs will not cause burning or pain.
    2. If the area to be treated has been frostbitten at any time or if the patient is hypersensitive to cold, use *extreme* caution or do not use cold at all.
    3. An undiagnosed or contagious skin rash is a contraindication for cold packs.
    4. If the area to be treated is sensitive to pressure, an instant pack is preferable to a large pack.

C. Keep the patient otherwise warm throughout the treatment.

D. Place one layer of a wet hand towel on the area to be treated.

E. Remove the pack from the cold pack unit or activate the pack.

F. Place the pack on the towel.

G. It may be necessary to use a second pack if the first pack is warm after ten minutes.

H. Treatment time is usually from ten to twenty minutes.

### *III. Terminating the Treatment*

A.  Remove the pack and towel from the patient.
B.  Check the patient's skin.

## Chapter 14

# PLASTIC BAG COLD PACKS

## *I. Preparations*

A.  Determine the procedure to be used:
   1. Plastic bag ice pack.
   2. Plastic bag slush pack.
B.  Ice pack:
   1. Fill a heavy plastic bag two-thirds full of ice:
      a. The plastic must be heavy to prevent tearing.
      b. The size should conform to the part being treated.
      c. Be sure the bag does not have any holes in it.
      d. Chipped, crushed ice or very small ice cubes will conform to the part more readily than will chunks of ice or regular size cubes.
   2. Remove as much air as possible, and seal the bag with an elastic band.
C.  Slush pack:
   1. Fill a heavy plastic bag two-thirds full of water and salt:
      a. The plastic must be heavy to prevent tearing.
      b. The size should conform to the part being treated.
      c. Be sure the bag does not have any holes in it.
      d. Add either one to two heaping tablespoons of salt to the water (depending on the size of the bag).
   2. Put the bag into a freezer for ten to twelve hours.
   3. The solution will not freeze solid but will remain pliable.
D.  Have sufficient towels ready as well as an extra drape sheet or cotton bath blanket to keep the patient warm.

## *II. Starting the Treatment*

A.  Explain the procedure to the patient:

1. Tell him why the pack is being used.
2. Tell him he should feel only a cold sensation.
3. Explain that a towel will be used between the pack and his skin to allow him to adjust to the cold gradually.
4. Assure him that the cold will not freeze the skin.
5. If he feels aching or numbness or any other discomfort, he should tell you.

B. Check the area to be treated:
   1. Skin sensation. The amount of skin sensation is usually of no importance as properly applied packs will not freeze the skin.
   2. If the area to be treated has been frostbitten at any time, use *extreme* caution or do not use cold at all.
   3. An undiagnosed or contagious skin disease is a contraindication to the use of the cold pack.

C. Check the patient's hypersensitivity to cold. This is a definite contraindication to cold on any part of the patient.
D. Keep the patient otherwise warm throughout the treatment.
E. Protect any remaining clothing from water.
F. Wrap the pack in a lukewarm damp towel so no more than one or two thicknesses of towel will be next to the patient.
G. Warn the patient and place the pack on the skin.
H. Cover the pack with a dry turkish towel to retard warming.
I. Hold the pack in place with a light sandbag, towels or straps.
J. The treatment time is usually five to twenty minutes.

### *III. Terminating the Treatment*

A. Remove the bag.
B. Give the patient a dry turkish towel and tell (help) him to dry himself.
C. Check the patient's skin.

*Chapter 15*

# VAPOR COOLANT SPRAYS

## *I. Preparations*

A.  Select the coolant:
   1. Fluori-Methane®:
      a. Nonflammable.
      b. Nontoxic when used correctly.
      c. Not explosive.
      d. Not a general anesthetic.
   2. Ethyl Chloride:
      a. Extremely flammable. Do *not* use near heat. *Never allow smoking in the same room.*
      b. Local anesthetic, and it is a general anesthetic when the vapor is inhaled.
      c. In certain concentrations with air, ethyl chloride is explosive.
B.  The container may deliver a jet stream or a fine spray. Usually a jet stream is needed for a small area.
C.  Have all necessary materials ready to use:
   1. Draping should be available:
      a. The patient's eyes must be protected from the vapor.
      b. The patient must be protected from possible inhalation of the vapor.
      c. Any exposed skin that is not going to be treated should be draped.
D.  Adequate ventilation and air movement in the room are important.

## *II. Starting the Treatment*

A.  Explain the procedure to the patient:
   1. Tell him the spray will feel cool/cold.
   2. If he feels an aching sensation, he should tell you.

131

3. Describe and demonstrate the stretching procedures you will do during the treatment.
4. Tell him his head/eyes/mouth will be covered to protect against inhalation of the vapor or damage to his eyes.

B. Check skin sensation. If sensation is lacking or diminished, use *extreme* caution.

C. Take care that you do not inhale the vapor and that your eyes are not affected.

D. Protect any skin not being treated.

E. Minimize inhalation of the vapor:
1. Elevate the head so it is above the level of the part being treated.
2. If treating the neck, face, shoulder or upper extremity, have the patient sit in a chair for treatment.
3. Cover the head.

F. During and after the spraying, gently stretch the involved muscle(s).

G. Technique for either coolant:
1. Do *not* frost the skin. If a white color appears on the skin, discontinue treatment.
2. Hold the container about 2 *feet* from the skin.
3. Apply the stream at an angle to the skin.
4. Start spraying at the point of pain and sweep outward from the trigger area. Do *not* sweep back and forth as in a painting motion.
5. Continue starting at the trigger point, and cover the entire area in rhythm of one or two seconds on and two or three seconds off.
6. If the patient complains of an aching sensation, lengthen the time between each sweep.
7. Continue spraying in this manner until the pain disappears or if there is no relief of pain after three or four minutes.
8. While you spray, gently stretch the involved muscle(s). The movement should be slow and without much force.
9. Repeat on other trigger areas if relief was evident after

the first area was treated.
10. Have the patient do simple and gentle exercises.

### III. Terminating the Treatment

A. Check the skin thoroughly for any unusual marks.

*Chapter 16*

# ICE MASSAGE

## *I. Preparations*

A.  Have the ice ready to use:
1. Water may be frozen in lightweight plastic or insulated cups:
   a. Medium size cups are better than small cups as they are easier to hold.
   b. Insulated cups protect the therapist's hand.
B.  Have towels and an extra drape sheet or cotton bath blanket ready to use.

## *II. Starting the Treatment*

A.  Explain the procedure to the patient:
1. Tell him why the ice is being used.
2. Describe the sensations he should expect to feel:
   a. The first sensation will be that of cold.
   b. Then he will experience a burning sensation.
   c. After approximately three minutes, he will feel an aching type of pain.
   d. In from.five to eight minutes, the skin should feel numb.
3. Ask the patient to tell you when he feels each of these sensations.
4. Reassure the patient that the treatment will not harm him in any way.
5. Tell him his skin should become red and have one or more white patches.
6. Tell him how long the treatment will be.
7. It may be necessary to let him feel the ice on another part of his body before starting treatment.
B.  Check skin sensation:

1. If skin sensation is lacking or diminished, use caution.
2. Do *not* use ice massage for longer than eight minutes. If the skin turns white before that time, stop the treatment.

C. Inspect the skin:
1. Do *not* use ice massage if an undiagnosed skin rash is present.
2. Do *not* massage over moles or warts.

D. Check the patient's hypersensitivity to cold:
1. Hypersensitivity is a contraindication to the use of ice massage on *any* part of the patient.
2. If the area to be treated has been frostbitten at any time, do *not* use ice massage on that area.

E. Keep the patient warm. Use an extra drape sheet, cotton bath blanket or towels.

F. Protect the patient, linen and any remaining clothing from water:
1. If treating the patient's back, shoulder or any area where the water will run off, use towels to prevent the melted water from running down the skin.
2. Use plastic or rubber sheeting with a towel on top of it to protect the plinth sheet.
3. Do *not* allow any of the patient's clothing to get wet.

G. Protect your hand from the ice:
1. If using ice in a cup, tear off the upper half of the cup and hold the ice in the bottom half.
2. If using an ice cube, wrap half of the cube in a face cloth, towel or gauze. When the wrapping becomes soaked, do not allow the water to drip on the patient.

H. Run the ice over your other hand so the rough edges will melt.

I. Warn the patient when you are about to put the ice on him. Do *not* take him by surprise.

J. Put the ice on his skin and start massaging immediately:
1. Take note of the time.
2. Use either a circular stroke or a back and forth movement.
3. The speed of the movement is about 2 inches per

second.

4. If treating a large area, divide it into sections no more than 6 inches in diameter, and massage each area separately.

5. Do *not* use heavy pressure. The weight of the ice alone is sufficient.

6. Avoid massaging over boney prominences.

K. The treatment time is usually five minutes or less. The massage should be stopped when the skin is white or at eight minutes, whichever comes first.

## III. Terminating the Treatment

A. Give the patient a dry turkish towel and instruct (help) him to dry himself.

B. Check the patient's skin.

C. Tell the patient the red color will dissipate.

*Chapter 17*

# EXTREMITY IMMERSION BATH

## *I. Preparations*

A. Set up the treatment where ice or cold water is available to maintain the proper water temperature.
B. You will need a container large enough to immerse the part to be treated. Large plastic or polyethylene wastebaskets may be used or whirlpool tanks with the turbine off.
C. Fill the clean container two-thirds full of water:
  1. The water temperature should be between 55° and 65° F.
  2. Do *not* fill the container too full as immersion of the extremity will cause the water to overflow.
  3. If the patient has an open or infected lesion, add some disinfectant.
D. Check the water temperature with a candy or dairy thermometer.
E. Turkish towels will be needed for drying the skin.

## *II. Starting the Treatment*

A. Be sure the patient is not hypersensitive to cold.
B. If treating the lower extremity:
  1. Provide a chair low (high) enough to allow the patient's foot to rest comfortably on the bottom of the container.
  2. Or the container may be elevated. Provide a footstool for the other foot.
  3. If using the leg whirlpool, hang the whirlpool seat in the water and have the patient rest the foot of the extremity to be treated on it.
C. Explain the procedure to the patient:
  1. The water is cold. Let him feel the water.

137

2. The extremity should be immersed *immediately* and *completely* into the water. The immersion should *not* be gradual.

3. If he cannot tolerate the cold or if any other untoward symptoms develop, he should tell you.

D. Instruct (help) the patient immerse the extremity.

E. Pad any pressure points.

F. The extremity should remain in the water until the part is relaxed or up to fifteen minutes:

   1. If spasticity is increased or if the patient cannot tolerate the cold, discontinue treatment.

   2. The patient may be able to tolerate the cold for only a few minutes initially.

G. The water temperature should be checked every few minutes. Add ice or cold water to maintain the correct temperature.

### III. Terminating the Treatment

A. Have (help) the patient remove the extremity and dry it thoroughly.

B. Check the skin.

C. Before allowing the patient to stand, wipe up any water from the floor.

D. Empty and clean the container.

### IV. Notes

A. The patient may be instructed to do the treatment at home:

   1. Tell him the water temperature.

   2. Tell him this temperature should be maintained throughout the treatment.

   3. Warn him about pressure points.

   4. Tell him how many times a day/week to use the cold.

# Part V
# Electricity Techniques

*Chapter 18*

# MEDICAL GALVANISM

## *I. Preparations*

A. Determine the procedure to be used:
   1. Select the unit. The unit must deliver *direct* current. Modulated direct current or alternating current *cannot* be used.
   2. Select the electrodes:
      a. Two electrodes will be needed.
      b. Usually electrodes of equal size and configuration are used. Electrode size determines the current density (concentration). The smaller the electrode, the greater the density and therefore, the patient will feel more current. Do *not* use electrodes smaller than 4 by 4 inches in size.
      c. If specific polarity effects are desired:
         1. The active electrode should be slightly smaller than the dispersive electrode.
         2. The polarity of both generator terminals *must* be known.
B. Check the current generator:
   1. Know how to operate the unit.
   2. All wire and plug connections should be tight.
   3. Do *not* use frayed conducting cords or electrode wires, corroded or loose-fitting electrode tips, etc.
   4. Use wire tips that fit both the electrodes and the unit. Substitutions or makeshift connections can cause burns.
   5. All controls should be off. Be especially certain that the intensity control is at zero.
   6. Turn on the main switch and warm up the unit if necessary. Most units that require warm-up will take

thirty seconds or less.

7. Try the current on yourself to be sure the unit is operating safely and efficiently.

C. Have all materials ready to use:
1. A wood plinth and/or table and wood chair are necessities. *Never* treat any part of a patient on a metal surface.
2. Warm water, or warm water to which salt has been added in which to soak the electrodes (not recommended).
3. Gauze or cotton to cover the electrodes for hygienic purposes.
4. Turkish towels.
5. Soak the electrodes in the warm water.

## II. Starting the Treatment

A. Explain the procedure to the patient:
1. Describe the sensation he should feel. It should be a gentle, prickly sensation that later changes to one of warmth. It may be necessary to demonstrate on yourself or let him feel the current.
2. Tell him not to move after the electrodes are in place, and tell him why.
3. Tell him not to touch/move the electrodes, wires, unit, or any metal, and explain why.
4. Emphasize that he should tell you *immediately* if he experiences any burning sensation or other discomfort.
5. Tell him the skin on the area will be red after treatment.

B. Inspect the area to be treated:
1. The skin should be clean and free from oils, creams, lotions, etc. as these are insulators against electricity.
2. Healing of cuts, abrasions, new skin and recent scar tissue may be enhanced by the electricity. However, a reduced intensity will be necessary because of the burning effect of the current. Avoid these areas if possible, or insulate them with dry gauze and a plastic or

rubber covering.

C. Check skin sensation. If sensation is lacking or diminished, use caution, and keep the intensity low:
  1. Try the current on another part of the patient. When he barely feels the prickly sensation, take note of the milliamperage and use the *same* intensity on the area to be treated.
  2. Or try the current on yourself.
  3. Frequently during the first treatment, slowly turn the intensity to zero, remove the electrodes and check the skin.
D. *Never* treat *any* part of *any* patient who has an external or implanted electrical or atomic stimulating device such as a pacemaker or transcutaneous nerve stimulator.
E. Do *not* treat through or around the heart.
F. Protect any remaining clothing from water.
G. Metal and medical galvanism:
  1. Remove all metal in or near the treatment area. Unremovable metal such as a wedding ring may be covered with a thick layer of dry gauze or cotton and covered with rubber or plastic.
  2. Any surface or superficially implanted metal is a contraindication for treatment in that area.
  3. If treating the face and the patient has fillings in his teeth, the patient may experience a metal taste. If the patient has braces on his teech, use caution.
  4. *Never* allow patients to touch a metal object such as the unit, a radiator, etc. at the same time they are being treated.
H. Remove the electrodes (sponges) from the water, and squeeze them very gently:
  1. The electrodes should be dripping wet. Too much water is better than too little.
  2. Keep the electrodes *soaked* during the treatment. *Slowly* turn the intensity to zero and add water when necessary.
  3. Cover each electrode with *wet* gauze for hygienic purposes:
    a. The gauze should be the *same* size as the electrode

pad or sponge. It should completely cover each electrode, but it should not be larger than the pad.

I. Connect the electrode wires to the electrodes.

J. Warn the patient.

K. Place the electrodes side by side (without touching) on the area to be treated, or place one electrode on the anterior (lateral) surface and the other on the posterior (medial) surface.

L. Firm (but not heavy) contact is essential. Use the patient's weight, light sandbags or straps to secure the electrodes.

M. Connect the electrode wires to the unit.

N. Recheck to be sure the electrodes are in good contact and will not slip off.

O. Cover the electrodes with a turkish towel to retard drying if they are not under the patient.

P. Recheck the unit:
   1. Be *sure* the intensity control is at zero.
   2. Polarity is of no concern.

Q. Turn on the unit. Allow for any warm-up time.

R. Warn the patient that you are about to turn on the current, and ask him to tell you when he barely begins to feel a prickly sensation. He will probably feel the prickle under the negative electrode first.

S. *Very slowly* turn up the intensity:
   1. If the patient feels nothing after increasing the intensity to .5 milliamperes, allow enough time for the current to overcome skin resistance, and then increase the intensity a little more. Continue to do this until the patient feels a prickly sensation.
   2. *Always* go by the patient's sensation (if normal). Do *not* increase the intensity beyond that which causes a slight prickly sensation.
   3. Approximately 1 milliampere of current per square inch of electrode surface should be sufficient.
   4. The prickly sensation may turn to one of warmth.

T. The intensity may have to be reduced after the first few minutes of treatment. Due to a breakdown of skin resistance, the milliamperage reading may be higher than the original setting, which indicates the patient is now getting more current. If this occurs, slowly reduce the intensity to the original setting.

U. Explain to the patient again that he should tell you *immediately* if any burning sensation, pain or other untoward symptoms develop. A burning sensation may mean the electrodes are too dry and/or the current intensity is too high.

V. Halfway through the treatment (unless treating for polarity effects):
   1. *Slowly* reduce the intensity to zero.
   2. Change the polarity either by means of the polarity switch or by switching the electrode wires.
   3. Resoak the electrodes if they need it.
   4. *Slowly* increase the intensity to the original meter setting.

W. Treatment time is usually twenty minues.

## III. Terminating the Treatment

A. *Slowly* reduce the intensity to zero and turn off the unit.
B. Remove the electrodes.
C. Move the unit to the back of the booth.
D. Instruct (help) the patient to dry himself thoroughly.
E. Check the patient's skin thoroughly for any unusual marks that were not there before treatment.
F. Tell the patient that the red skin color will disappear in an hour or less, but if he takes a warm bath or puts the extremity in warm water, the redness may return.
G. Record the intensity used.

## Chapter 19

# IONTOPHORESIS

## I. Preparations

A. Determine the procedure to be used:
  1. Select the unit to be used. The unit must deliver direct current. Alternating current or modulated direct current cannot be used.
B. Check the current generator:
  1. Know how to operate the unit.
  2. The polarity of both generator terminals *must* be known.
  3. All wire and plug connections should be tight.
  4. Do *not* use frayed conducting cords or electrode wires, corroded or loose-fitting electrode tips, etc.
  5. Use wire tips that fit both the electrodes and the unit. Substitutions or makeshift connections can cause burns.
  6. All controls should be off. Be especially certain that the intensity control is at zero.
  7. Turn on the main switch and warm up the unit if necessary.
  8. Try the current on yourself to be sure the unit is operating safely and efficiently.
C. Select the technique to be used:
  1. If using a solution, a pad will be needed to hold the solution:
    a. Asbestos paper, blotting paper, a cloth hand towel, gauze or cotton at least 1/2 inch thick may be used.
    b. The solution pad should be the *same* size as the area to be treated but larger than the active electrode.
    c. The pad must *not* have any holes or very thin areas in it. Be especially careful of asbestos or blotting

146

paper.
    d. A flexible metal plate may be used as the active electrode:
        1. This plate must be *smaller* than the solution pad.
        2. One electrode wire will require a clamp tip to connect it to the metal plate.
  2. If using an ointment, the ointment is usually rubbed into the skin and then a pad electrode is used as the active electrode on the ointment:
    a. The pad electrode should be the *same* size as the area being treated.
    b. If the area to be treated is large, divide it into sections and treat each area separately.
    c. Soak the pad electrode in warm water.
D. Drug polarity *must* be known:
  1. Drug ions that carry a positive charge require that the active electrode be positive.
  2. Drug ions that carry a negative charge require that the active electrode be negative.
E. Dispersive electrode for either technique:
  1. The dispersive electrode should be at least 5 by 7 inches in size and preferably larger.
  2. Soak the electrode in warm water.
F. Have all other materials ready to use:
  1. A wood plinth and/or table, wood chair. *Never* treat any part of any patient on a metal surface.
  2. Turkish towels.
  3. Gauze to cover the electrodes for hygienic purposes.


## II. Starting the Treatment

A. If possible, determine the patient's sensitivity to the drug.
B. Explain the procedure to the patient:
  1. Describe the sensation he should feel. It should be a gently prickly sensation that later turns to one of warmth.
  2. Tell the patient not to move after the electrodes are in place and tell him why.

3. Emphasize that he should tell you *immediately* if he experiences any burning sensation or other discomfort.
4. Tell the patient that the skin on the treated area may be red after treatment.
5. It may be necessary to let him feel the current on another part of his body before treating him.

C. Inspect the area to be treated:
   1. The skin should be clean and free from oils, creams, lotions, etc. as these are insulators against current.
   2. Do *not* treat over abrasions, cuts, new skin or recent scar tissue. Small areas may be padded with *dry* gauze and covered with plastic or rubber to insulate them against the current.

D. Check skin sensation. If sensation is lacking or diminished, use caution and keep the intensity low:
   1. Try the current on another part of the patient. When he barely begins to feel the prickly sensation, take note of the milliamperage and use that *same* intensity on the area to be treated.
   2. Or try the current on yourself.
   3. Frequently during the first treatment, slowly turn the intensity control to zero, remove the electrodes and check the skin.

E. *Never* treat *any* part of *any* patient who has an external or implanted electrical or atomic stimulating device such as a heart pacemaker or transcutaneous nerve stimulator.

F. Do *not* treat through or around the heart.

G. Protect any remaining clothing from water.

H. Metal and iontophoresis:
   1. Remove all metal in or near the treatment area. Unremovable metal, such as rings, is a contraindication for treatment on that area.
   2. Any surface or superficially implanted metal is a contraindication for treating in that area.
   3. If treating the face and the patient has metal fillings in his teeth, he may experience an "aluminum" taste. If the patient has braces on his teeth, use caution.
   4. *Never* allow the patient to touch a metal object such as

the unit, a table, radiator, etc. at the same time he is being treated.

I. Solution pad technique:
1. The solution strength should be 1 percent or less.
2. If you are sensitive to the solution, wear rubber gloves.
3. Soak the pad in the solution.
4. Squeeze the pad gently, but do not wring. The pad should be thoroughly soaked and not merely damp.
5. Spread out the pad, being careful not to tear any holes in it.
6. Warn the patient and place the pad on the skin.
7. Place the *smaller* flexible metal plate on the pad:
    a. Absolutely *no* part of the metal plate may touch the patient's skin.
    b. Firm and complete contact is essential. Use light sandbag, the patient's weight or a strap to hold the electrode securely in place.

J. Ointment technique:
1. The ointment strength should be 1 percent or less.
2. If you are sensitive to the drug, wear rubber gloves.
3. Use cotton or gauze to rub the ointment into the skin:
    a. Warn the patient before applying the ointment.
    b. The ointment should cover the entire area to be treated.
4. A regular pad electrode or one with a sponge insert may be used as the active electrode:
    a. It should be the same size as the area to be treated. If the area is too large, divide it into sections and treat each section separately.
    b. Soak the electrode in warm water and squeeze gently to remove excess water.
    c. Cover the pad (sponge) with several layers of wet gauze.
    d. Warn the patient, and place the electrode on the ointment. Firm and complete contact is essential. Use light sandbags, the patient's weight or a strap to hold the electrode securely in place.
    e. This electrode (sponge) must be washed thoroughly

　　　with soap and water after each treatment to remove any traces of the ointment.

K. Dispersive electrode for either technique:
　　1. This electrode should be at least 5 by 7 inches in size.
　　2. Remove the electrode from the warm water.
　　3. Squeeze gently to remove excess water. Too much water is better than too little.
　　4. Cover the electrode with wet gauze for hygienic purposes. The gauze covering should be the same size as the electrode (sponge).
　　5. Warn the patient and place the electrode on the *same* side (left versus right) of the patient as that being treated. (Example: The right anterior thigh is being treated. Place the dispersive electrode under the right thigh. If treating the back, place the electrode under a thigh.)
　　6. Firm and complete contact is essential. Use the patient's body weight, a light sandbag or a strap to hold the electrode securely in place.

L. Connect the electrode wires to the electrodes and to the unit.

M. Recheck to be sure the electrodes are in good contact and will not slip off if the patient moves.

N. Recheck the unit:
　　1. The correct polarity *must* be used or the treatment will be ineffective. If the drug ions are positive, the active electrode must be attached to the positive pole of the unit.
　　2. Be *sure* the intensity control is at zero.
　　3. Turn on the unit.

O. Warn the patient that you are about to turn on the current, and ask him to tell you when he barely begins to feel a prickly sensation.

P. *Very slowly* turn up the intensity in increment steps:
　　1. Turn the intensity to 1 milliampere and stop. If the patient feels nothing, increase the intensity to 2 milliamperes. Continue until the patient feels the current (unless sensation is impaired). One half to 1 milliam-

pere of current per each square inch of the active electrode surface is usually sufficient.

2. Always go by the patient's sensation if normal.
3. Impress upon the patient that a little sensation is sufficient.
4. The prickly sensation may turn to one of warmth after a few minutes.
5. The intensity may have to be reduced after four or five minutes due to the breakdown of skin resistance.

Q. Check the electrodes after ten minutes to be sure they are both secure and as moist as they should be.
R. Treatment time is usually twenty minutes.

### III. Terminating the Treatment

A. *Slowly* turn the intensity control to zero.
B. Turn off the unit.
C. Remove the electrodes.
D. Instruct (help) the patient to wash off his skin.
E. Thoroughly check the patient's skin.

*Chapter 20*

# ELECTRICAL STIMULATION

## Unipolar Technique

### *I. Preparations*

A. Select the current:
    1. If a muscle is completely denervated, a modulated (interrupted, surged) direct current *must* be used.
    2. Alternating current may be used to stimulate muscles weak from disuse.

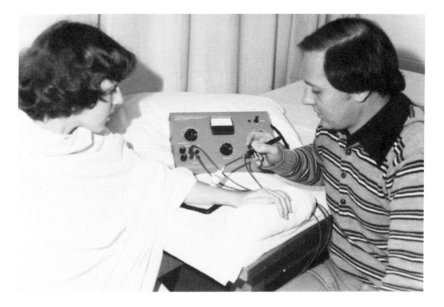

Figure 32. Unipolar technique. (Teca Corp. Sp2)

B. The unipolar technique (electrodes of unequal size):
    1. This technique may be used with either modulated direct current or alternating current.
    2. Unless the active electrode is the same size as the

muscle, this technique supplies current to only part of the muscle.

    3. This technique must be used when the muscles are too small to use the bipolar technique or when trying to elicit a contraction of only one muscle.

C. The active electrode:

    1. The active electrode is smaller than the dispersive electrode.

    2. The electrodes vary in size and shape. They may be round metal discs, bare screw heads or square or rectangular pieces of metal.

    3. Any bare metal *must always* be completely covered by a pad of gauze or cotton unless padding is provided by the manufacturer.

    4. The electrodes can be or are attached to a handle. The handle may have a make and break key or it may have a voltage regulator.

    5. A commercial electrode pad should be covered with gauze for hygienic reasons:

        a. Hold the covering in place with an elastic band.

        b. Any loose ends should be included under the elastic band to prevent them from touching the patient as they provide unwanted pathways for the current.

    6. Place the electrode in warm water to soak.

D. The dispersive (indifferent) electrode:

    1. The dispersive electrode is larger than the active electrode.

    2. These electrodes vary in size and shape. They may be 1 by 1 inch up to 8 by 10 inch squares, rectangles or circles. A large dispersive electrode is preferable to a small one.

    3. Any bare metal *must always* be completely covered with a pad of gauze or cotton at least 1/4 inch thick unless padding is provided by the manufacturer.

    4. Place the electrode in warm water to soak.

E. Have all other necessary materials ready to use:

    1. Wood plinth and chair. *Never* treat any part of the patient on a metal surface.

    2. Turkish towels.

    3. Motor point charts if necessary.

F.  Check the unit to be used:
1. Know how to operate the unit.
2. All wire and plug connections should be tight.
3. Do *not* use frayed conducting cords or electrode wires, corroded or loose-fitting wire tips.
4. Use wire tips that fit both the unit and the electrodes. Substitutions or makeshift connections can cause burns.
5. All controls should be off. Be especially certain that the intensity control is at zero.
6. Turn on the main switch and warm up the unit if necessary. Most units that require warm-up will take thirty seconds or less.
7. Try the current on yourself to be sure the unit is operating safely and efficiently.

## II. Starting the Treatment

A.  Explain the procedure to the patient:
1. Describe the sensation he should feel. Do not scare the patient. Use positive terms.
2. Tell him what the electricity will do and why it is being used.
3. Explain that you will need to use only a small amount of current.
4. *Demonstrate on yourself.* Get an actual contraction; don't fake it.
5. It may be necessary to let him feel the current before you treat him.
6. Tell him the skin on the treated area may be red after treatment.

B.  The skin should be clean and free from oils, creams, lotions, etc. as these are insulators against electricity.

C.  Check skin sensation. If sensation is lacking or diminished, use caution. To determine the intensity that will be needed when sensation is not normal:
1. Try the current on another part of the patient (if sensa-

tion is normal) and get the same amount of muscle contraction you will use for treatment. Note the milli-amperage and use that same intensity on the muscle(s) to be stimulated, or

2. Try the current on yourself.

D. *Never* treat *any* part of *any* patient who has an external or implanted electrical or atomic stimulating device such as a cardiac pacemaker.

E. Do *not* stimulate:
  1. Directly over, through or in the vicinity of the heart.
  2. Any part of any patient who has a coronary problem.
  3. Directly over, through or near a recent or nonunion fracture.
  4. On old scar tissue as it offers a great deal of resistance to current.
  5. Over, near or through a pregnant uterus.
  6. On cuts, abrasions, new skin, recent scar tissue, etc. Although healing may be enhanced by the electricity, a reduced intensity will be necessary. Therefore, the intensity may not be sufficient to cause a muscle contraction. Avoid these areas or insulate them with thick pads of dry gauze and a plastic or rubber covering over the gauze.
  7. Moles, warts, etc.

F. Metal and electrical stimulation:
  1. Always use a wood plinth/chair/table.
  2. Remove all metal in or near the area to be treated. Any unremovable metal, such as a wedding ring, may be covered with a thick pad of dry gauze or cotton and covered with a piece of plastic or rubber.
  3. Any implanted metal that is near the surface should be avoided.
  4. If stimulating the face and the patient has metal fillings or is wearing braces, he will probably experience a metal taste.
  5. *Never* allow the patient to touch a metal object, such as the unit, a radiator, etc. at the same time he is being treated.

G. *Check the patient's voluntary motion:*
   1. If he can voluntarily contract a muscle, use alternating current.
   2. You *must* use modulated direct current if the muscle is completely denervated.
   3. If the muscle is extremely weak, modulated direct current may elicit a better contraction with less intensity than will alternating current.
H. If the patient's skin is colder than the room temperature, preheating the skin with an infrared lamp, hot packs or whirlpool for five minutes will reduce skin resistance:
   1. Reduced skin resistance requires less intensity.
   2. The paraffin bath may *not* be used, because the oil left on the skin will act as an insulator against the current.
   3. It is not necessary to use deep heat.
I. Protect any remaining clothing and the linen from the water.
J. Dispersive electrode:
   1. Remove the dispersive electrode from the water.
   2. New or completely dried out pad electrodes will require up to twenty minutes soaking.
   3. The electrode *must* be soaked all the way through.
   4. Cover the pad (sponge) with several layers of gauze for hygienic purposes. The gauze should cover the pad/ sponge, but it should not be larger than the electrode.
   5. Squeeze the electrode gently to remove the excess water. Too much water is better than too little. Both the pad and the gauze should be dripping wet.
   6. Keep the electrode soaked throughout the treatment.
   7. Attach a lead wire to the electrode and to the unit. This electrode is usually connected to the *positive* terminal when using modulated direct current.
   8. Warn the patient, and then place the electrode on his skin:
      a. *Firm* and *complete* contact is *essential.* The patient's body weight, light sandbags or straps may be used to maintain excellent contact.
      b. The electrode is usually placed on the *same* side of

the body as that being treated.

K. Active electrode:
  1. Remove the electrode from the water. (It should already have been covered with a hygienic covering.)
  2. The electrode *must* be wet all the way through.
  3. Gently squeeze out the excess water. Too much water is better than too little.
  4. The electrode should be dipped in water frequently during the treatment to keep it soaked.
  5. Attach a lead wire to the electrode and to the unit:
     a. The active electrode is usually connected to the *negative* pole if using modulated direct current.
     b. The lead wire must be connected to the correct outlet on the electrode handle:
        1. If the make and break key is to be used as it has to be with direct current or continuous tetanizing current, connect the wire to this outlet.
        2. If the unit is to control the current modulations, connect the wire to the other terminal or hold down the make and break key.
  6. Warn the patient, and place the electrode in *firm* but not heavy contact on the muscle to be stimulated:
     a. When the muscle is denervated, place the electrode on the distal end of the muscle belly toward the tendon of insertion (or on the tendon of insertion if no contraction can be elicited on the muscle belly).
     b. If the muscle is innervated, the electrode should be placed on the motor point.
L. Recheck to be sure the intensity control is at zero, and then turn on the unit, unless it has been warming.
M. When everything is ready, warn the patient that you are about to turn on the current. Do *not* take him by surprise.
N. If using the make and break key, correct and excellent technique is essential:
  1. Turn up the intensity slightly, press the key and release it *immediately*. The shorter the time the key is down, the less will be the sensory effects.
  2. When locating the motor point or most active area,

stimulate at least *four* times in the *same* place to break down skin resistance *before* increasing the intensity.

3. Keep the electrode in the *same* place, increase the intensity slightly and stimulate four times.
4. Move the electrode to another spot and repeat.
5. Keep moving the electrode, adjusting the intensity and stimulating at least four times until the most excitable area is found.
5. When the motor point or most active area has been located it may be necessary to reduce the intensity. *Get the best contraction with the least intensity.*

O. *Before* stimulating another muscle or when increasing the frequency of alternating current, *reduce* the intensity to zero.

P. It is *not* necessary to produce joint motion.

Q. Usually, ten to twenty muscle contractions are sufficient before moving to another muscle:
   1. Avoid overstimulation. Very weak and denervated muscles will tire quickly.
   2. If the skin becomes excessively red, change to another muscle.

R. In order to elicit a good muscle contraction with the least amount of current intensity, the following must occur simultaneously:
   1. The electrodes *must* be wet enough.
   2. The active electrode *must* be on the motor point or the most active area.
   3. The intensity *must* be high enough.
   4. The duration of the current impulse *must* be long enough.
   5. The rate of rise to rheobase *must* be fast enough.

### III. Terminating the Treatment

A. If the unit is modulating the current, *slowly* decrease the intensity to zero; or remove the active electrode during a break in the current.

B. Turn off the unit.

C. Remove the electrodes.
D. Instruct (help) the patient dry himself thoroughly.
E. Check the patient's skin for any unusual marks.
F. Tell the patient the red skin color should disappear, but it may reappear if he takes a warm bath (if modulated direct current has been used).

## BIPOLAR TECHNIQUE

### *I. Preparations*

A. Select the current:
 1. If a muscle is completely denervated, a modulated (interrupted, surged) direct current *must* be used.

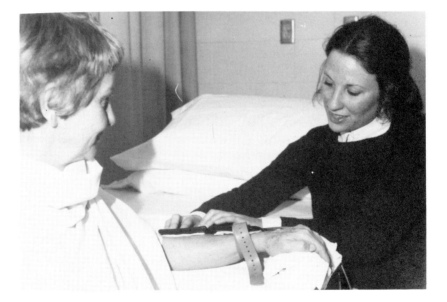

Figure 33. Bipolar technique.

 2. Alternating current may be used to stimulate muscles weak from disuse.
B. Bipolar technique (electrodes of equal size and configuration):
 1. This technique is used to stimulate the entire muscle or

a muscle group.

2. Any bare metal *must* always be completely covered by a pad of gauze or cotton at least 1/4 inch thick unless padding is provided by the manufacturer.

3. Two or four electrodes of equal size and shape may be used at the same time. No one electrode should touch another electrode.

4. If using two electrodes, there are several methods of placement:
   a. Place both electrodes on the same muscle (one on each end of the muscle belly) or on the same muscle group.
   b. If the electrodes are small, place one electrode on the motor point or the distal end of the muscle belly toward the tendon of insertion, and the other electrode on the opposite end of the muscle belly.

5. If using four electrodes:
   a. Place all four electrodes on the anterior (lateral) surface such as the quadriceps and the other two electrodes on the posterior (medial) surface such as the hamstrings.

C. Have all other materials ready to use:
   1. Wood plinth and chair. *Never* treat any part of the patient on a metal surface.
   2. Turkish towels.
   3. Motor point charts if necessary.

D. Check the unit:
   1. Know how to operate the unit.
   2. All wire and plug connections should be tight.
   3. Do *not* use frayed conducting cords or electrode wires, corroded or loose-fitting wire tips.
   4. Use wire tips that fit both the unit and the electrodes. Substitutions or makeshift connections can cause burns.
   5. All controls should be off. Be especially certain that the intensity control is at zero.
   6. Turn on the main switch and warm up the unit if necessary. Most units that require warm-up will take

thirty seconds or less.

7. Try the current on yourself to be sure the unit is operating safely and efficiently.

## II. Starting the Treatment

A. Explain the procedure to the patient:
   1. Describe the sensation he should feel. Do not scare the patient. Use positive terms.
   2. Tell him what the electricity will do and why it is being used.
   3. Explain that you will need to use only a small amount of current.
   4. *Demonstrate on yourself.* Get an actual contraction; don't fake it!
   5. It may be necessary to let him feel the current before you treat him.
   6. Tell him the skin on the treated area may be red after treatment.
B. The skin should be clean and free from oils, lotions, and creams, etc. as these are insulators against electricity.
C. Check skin sensation. If sensation is lacking or diminished, use caution. To determine the intensity that will be needed when sensation is not normal:
   1. Try the current on another part of the patient (if sensation is normal) and get the same amount of muscle contraction (reaction) you will use for treatment. Note the milliamperage and use that same intensity on muscle(s) to be stimulated, or
   2. Try the current on yourself.
D. *Never* treat *any* part of *any* patient who has an external or implanted electrical or atomic stimulating device such as a cardiac pacemaker.
E. Do *not* stimulate:
   1. Directly over, through or in the vicinity of the heart.
   2. Any part of any patient who has a coronary problem.
   3. Directly over, through or near a recent or nonunion fracture.

4. On old scar tissue as it offers a great deal of resistance to current.

5. Over, near or through a pregnant uterus.

6. On cuts, abrasions, new skin, recent scar tissue, etc. Although healing may be enhanced by electricity, a reduced intensity will be necessary. Therefore, the intensity may not be sufficient to cause a muscle contraction. Avoid these areas or insulate them with thick pads of dry gauze and a plastic or rubber covering over the gauze.

7. Moles, warts, etc.

F.  Metal and electrical stimulation:

1. Always use a wood plinth/chair/table.

2. Remove all metal in or near the area to be treated. Any unremovable metal, such as a wedding ring, may be covered with a thick pad of dry gauze or cotton and covered with a piece of plastic or rubber.

3. Any implanted metal that is near the surface should be insulated or avoided.

4. Never allow the patient to touch a metal object, such as the unit, a radiator, etc. at the same time he is being treated.

G.  *Check the patient's voluntary motion:*

1. If he can voluntarily contract a muscle, use alternating current.

2. You *must* use modulated direct current if the muscle is completely denervated.

3. If the muscle is extremely weak, modulated direct current may elicit a better muscle contraction with less intensity than will alternating current.

H.  If the patient's skin is colder than the room temperature, preheating the skin with an infrared lamp, hot packs or whirlpool for five minutes will reduce skin resistance:

1. Reduced skin resistance requires less intensity.

2. The paraffin bath may *not* be used because the oil left on the skin will act as an insulator against the current.

3. It is not necessary to use deep heat.

I.  Protect any remaining clothing and the linen from the

water.

J. Cover each electrode with several thicknesses of gauze for hygienic purposes:
1. The gauze should be the same size as the electrodes.
2. The gauze should completely cover the electrode, but it should not be larger than the electrode.

K. Soak the electrodes and gauze in warm water:
1. The electrodes must be wet all the way through.
2. Keep the electrodes soaked throughout the treatment.

L. Squeeze each electrode gently to remove the excess water:
1. Do not squeeze dry. Both the electrode and the gauze should be dripping wet.

M. Attach lead wires to each electrode and to the unit.

N. Warn the patient that you are about to place the electrodes onto his skin.

O. Position the electrodes:
1. Good contact is essential.
2. Hold the electrodes in place with straps, sandbags or with your hand:
    a. If using alternating current, the electrodes are sometimes left in place for twenty minutes.
    b. If the muscles are extremely weak or denervated, the electrodes will have to be moved often.

P. Recheck to be sure the intensity control is at zero, and then turn on the unit, unless it has been warming.

Q. When everything is ready, warn the patient that you are about to turn on the current. Do *not* take him by surprise.

R. *Slowly* increase the current intensity until a muscle contraction is observed. Get the best contraction with the least amount of current intensity.

S. In order to elicit a good muscle contraction with the least amount of current, the following must occur simultaneously:
1. The electrodes *must* be soaking wet.
2. The intensity must be high enough.
3. The duration of the current impulse must be long enough.
4. The rate of rise of the current from zero to rheobase

intensity must be fast enough.

### III. Terminating the Treatment

A.  If the unit is modulating the current, *slowly* decrease the intensity to zero.
B.  Turn off the unit.
C.  Remove the electrodes.
D.  Give the patient a dry turkish towel and instruct (help) him to dry himself thoroughly.
E.  Check the patient's skin for any unusual marks.
F.  The red skin color will disappear, but may reappear if the patient takes a warm bath/shower (if modulated DC has been used).

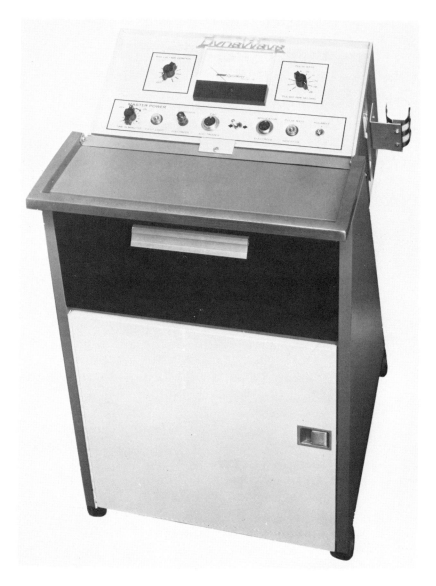

Figure 34. Dynawave electrical stimulation unit. (Courtesy of Dynawave Corp.)

## Chapter 21

# ELECTRICAL TESTING

## Strength-Duration Test
## Chronaxic Meter®: Teca Corporation

### *I. Preparations*

A. Determine the procedure to be used:
1. Select the unit:
   a. The unit must deliver direct current that can be interrupted manually or automatically by the unit.
   b. The unit must have a pulse duration switch to control the length of time the current is on. Desirable durations are from .05 milliseconds to at least 100 milliseconds.
2. Select the stimulation technique:
   a. The unipolar technique is the technique of choice (see Chap. 20).
   b. The therapist should be skilled in electrical stimulation to assure accurate results.
3. Select the electrodes:
   a. The active electrode should be small enough to stimulate the muscle to be tested and to limit current overflow as much as possible.
   b. The dispersive electrode should be at least 4 by 4 inches in size.
B. Have all materials ready to use:
1. Wood plinth. Do not use a metal plinth or table.
2. Warm water in which to soak the electrodes.
3. Turkish towels.
4. Record forms.
C. Check the unit to be used:
1. Know how to operate the unit.
2. All wire and plug connections should be tight.
3. Do *not* use frayed conducting cords or electrode wires,

corroded or loose-fitting wire tips, etc.
  4. Use wire tips that fit both the unit and the electrodes. Substitutions or makeshift connections can cause burns.
  5. All controls should be off. Be especially certain that the intensity control is off.
  6. Soak the electrodes in warm water.
  7. Turn on the main switch and warm up the unit if necessary. Some units will require five minutes to warm up.
  8. Try the current on yourself to be sure the unit is safe.
D.  Type of muscle contraction:
  1. The minimal perceptible response (MPR) should be used. This is a *flicker* of the muscle or tendon of insertion that can barely be seen.

## II. Starting the Test

A.  Explain the procedure to the patient:
  1. Describe the sensation he should feel. Use positive terms.
  2. Tell him what the electricity will do and why the test is being done.
  3. Explain that you will need to use only a small amount of current.
  4. *Demonstrate on yourself.* Get an actual contraction; don't fake it.
  5. It may be necessary to let him feel the current before you start the test.
  6. Assure him that the test is completely safe.
  7. Tell him that the skin on the test area will be red.
B.  Inspect the area to be tested:
  1. The skin should be clean and free from oils, creams, and lotions as these are insulators against electricity.
  2. Avoid stimulating on cuts, abrasions, moles, new skin, recent scar tissue, etc.
C.  Check skin sensation. If sensation is lacking or diminished, use caution.

D. *Never* stimulate *any* part of *any* patient who has an external or implanted electrical or atomic stimulating device such as a heart pacemaker.
E. Do *not* stimulate:
   1. Directly through, over or in the area of the heart.
   2. Any part of any patient who has a coronary problem.
   3. Directly over, through or near a recent or nonunion fracture site.
   4. On old scar tissue, as it offers a great deal of resistance to current.
   5. Over, near, or through a pregnant uterus.
F. Metal and electrical testing:
   1. Always use a wood plinth or table and chair.
   2. Remove all metal in the area to be tested. Any unremovable metal, such as a wedding ring, may be covered with a thick pad of dry gauze and plastic or rubber.
   3. Do *not* allow the patient to touch any metal while he is being tested.
G. Reduce skin resistance. Skin resistance will require more intensity to elicit the minimal perceptible response. Reduce skin resistance by:
   1. Initially soaking the electrodes and keeping them soaked throughout the test.
   2. Stimulating at least four times in the same place.
   3. Warming the skin with mild heat such as that from an infrared lamp, hot packs or whirlpool if the skin is cold. Do not use a deep heating unit or paraffin.
H. Protect any remaining clothing from the water.
I. Dispersive electrode:
   1. Remove the electrode (sponge) from the water.
   2. Cover the electrode with several layers of gauze or cotton for hygienic purposes. The gauze should completely cover the electrode pad, but it should not be larger than the pad.
   3. Squeeze the electrode and gauze gently to remove excess water. The electrode should be wet and not damp. Too much water is better than too little.
   4. Attach a lead wire to the electrode and to the unit.

5. Warn the patient.
6. Place the electrode in *firm* and *complete* contact on the *same* side (left versus right) as the muscle you will test, but on a different surface:
   a. Use the patient's weight, light sandbags, or straps to hold the electrode securely.
   b. The electrode should remain in the *same* place throughout the test.
   c. For subsequent tests on the same muscle(s), the dispersive electrode should be in *exactly* the *same* place as for the first test.
7. The dispersive electrode should be *positive.*

J. Active electrode:
1. This electrode should be *negative.*
2. Remove the electrode from the water.
3. Cover the electrode with several layers of gauze for hygienic purposes:
   a. Hold the gauze in place with an elastic band.
   b. Any loose ends should be included under the elastic band to prevent them from touching the patient.
4. Attach a lead wire to the electrode and to the unit:
   a. Use the correct wire tips. Substitutions or makeshift connections can cause burns.
   b. When the make and break key is used, be sure to connect the lead wire to the correct terminal on the handle.
5. Recheck to be sure the intensity control is at zero, and then turn on the unit (unless preheated).
6. Warn the patient.
7. Place the electrode in *firm* but not heavy contact on the muscle to be tested.
8. Find the area of maximum irritability and *stay on it throughout the test.*

K. Set Selector to CHRON.
L. The intensity should be off.
M. Set the Pulse Interval to 0.5 seconds.
N. Set the Pulse Duration to 100 or 300 milliseconds.
O. Find the intensity sufficient to cause a minimal perceptible

# ELECTRODIAGNOSTIC TEST

Date _____

Name _____ Age _____ Tested by _____

Address or Ward _____ Sex _____ Inst. No. _____

History _____

_____

_____

————————— CHRONAXIE —————————

|  | | MUSCLE | | MUSCLE | | MUSCLE | |
|---|---|---|---|---|---|---|---|
| DURATION DIAL SETTING | MAIN | L | R | L | R | | R |
| | VERNIER | | | | | | |
| | MULTIPLIER | | | | | | |
| CHRONAXIE | | | | | | | |

————————— STRENGTH DURATION CURVE ————— INTERVAL _____ SEC.

| PULSE DURATION MILLISEC. | MUSCLE | | MUSCLE | | MUSCLE | |
|---|---|---|---|---|---|---|
| | CURRENT | NOTES | CURRENT | NOTES | CURRENT | NOTES |
| 100 | | | | | | |
| 70 | | | | | | |
| 50 | | | | | | |
| 30 | | | | | | |
| 10 | | | | | | |
| 7 | | | | | | |
| 5 | | | | | | |
| 3 | | | | | | |
| 2 | | | | | | |
| 1 | | | | | | |
| 0.8 | | | | | | |
| 0.6 | | | | | | |
| 0.4 | | | | | | |
| 0.3 | | | | | | |
| 0.1 | | | | | | |
| .05 | | | | | | |

ADDITIONAL TESTS _____

_____

_____

_____

**Teca Corp. Form ET-3 B**

Figure 35. Electrodiagnostic test record. (Courtesy of Teca Corp.)

response (MPR).

P. Record the pulse duration and milliameter readings.
Q. Repeat the test after decreasing the Pulse Duration to 100 or less milliseconds, and record findings.
R. Continue to decrease the pulse duration in steps as indicated on the record form.
S. Readjust the intensity to obtain the *same* amount of MPR.
T. Plot the intensity readings on the record form, and then connect the dots to show the strength-duration curve.

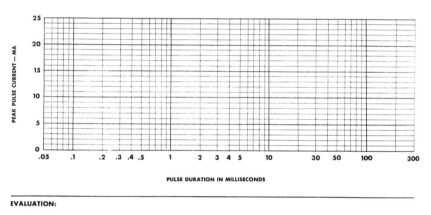

Figure 36. Strength-duration curve plotting record. (Courtesy of Teca Corp.)

## III. Terminating the Test

A. Decrease the intensity to zero.
B. Remove the electrodes.
C. Give the patient a dry turkish towel and tell (help) him to dry his skin.
D. Turn off the unit and move it out of the patient's way.
E. Check the patient's skin.
F. Advise the patient that the redness will disappear but it may come back if he takes a bath or shower.

## REACTION OF DEGENERATION

### *I. Preparations*

A. Determine the procedure to be used:
   1. Select the unit:
     a. The unit must deliver either direct current that can be interrupted manually or automatically by the unit, and it must deliver continuous alternating current at 100 cycles per second, or two different units may be used.
   2. Select the stimulation technique:
     a. The unipolar technique is the technique of choice (see Chap. 20).
     b. The therapist should be skilled in electrical stimulation to assure accurate test results.
   3. Select the electrodes:
     a. The active electrode should be small enough to stimulate the muscle to be tested and to limit current overflow as much as possible.
     b. The dispersive electrode should be at least 4 by 4 inches in size.
B. Have all materials ready to use:
   1. Wood plinth or table and chair.
   2. Warm water for soaking the electrodes.
   3. Motor point charts.
   4. Record forms.
   5. Turkish towels.
C. Check the unit to be used:
   1. Know how to operate the unit.
   2. All wire and plug connections should be tight.
   3. Do *not* use frayed conducting cords or electrode wires, corroded or loose-fitting wire tips, etc.
   4. Use wire tips that fit both the unit and the electrodes. Substitutions or makeshift connections can cause burns.
   5. All controls should be off. Be especially certain that the intensity control is off.

6. Soak the electrodes in the warm water.
7. Turn on the main switch and warm up the unit if necessary. Most units that require warm-up will take thirty seconds or less, but check the manufacturer's directions.
8. Try the currents on yourself to be sure the unit is operating safely and efficiently.

D. Type of muscle contraction:
   1. You will need to use enough intensity to produce a strong muscle contraction.
      a. Do not cause pain.
      b. There is no need to cause joint motion.

## II. Starting the Test

A. Explain the procedure to the patient:
   1. Describe the sensation he should feel. Use positive terms.
   2. Tell him what the electricity will do and why the test is being done.
   3. Explain that you will need to use only a small amount of current.
   4. *Demonstrate on yourself.* Get an actual contraction; don't fake it.
   5. Assure him that the test is completely safe.
   6. Tell him that his skin may be red.
   7. It may be necessary to let him feel the current on another part of his body before the test is done.
B. Inspect the area(s) to be tested:
   1. The skin should be clean and free from oils, lotions and creams.
   2. Avoid stimulating on abrasions, new skin, recent scar tissue, moles, etc.
C. Check skin sensation. If sensation is lacking or diminished, use caution.
D. *Never* stimulate *any* part of *any* patient who has an external or implanted electrical or atomic stimulating device such as a heart pacemaker or transcutaneous nerve stimula-

tion unit.

E. Do *not* stimulate:
1. Directly through, over or near a recent or nonunion fracture.
2. Directly through, over or in the vicinity of the heart.
3. Any part of any patient who has a coronary problem.
4. Directly through, over or near a pregnant uterus.
5. On old scar tissue as it offers a great deal of resistance to current.

F. Metal and electrical testing:
1. Always use a wood plinth or table and chair.
2. Remove all metal in the area to be tested. Any unremovable metal, such as a wedding ring, may be covered with a thick pad of dry cotton or gauze and then covered with plastic or rubber.
3. Do *not* allow the patient to touch any metal while he is being tested.

G. Skin resistance will require more intensity to elicit the MPR. Reduce skin resistance by:
1. Initially soaking the electrodes and keeping them soaked throughout the test.
2. Stimulating at least four times in the same place.
3. Warming the skin with mild heat from an infrared lamp, hot packs or a whirlpool before the test if the skin is cold.

H. Protect any remaining clothing and sheets from the water.

I. Check the patient's voluntary motion:
1. Ask the patient to voluntarily contract the involved muscle(s) you are going to test.
2. If there is no voluntary motion, proceed with the test.

J. Begin with the *same* muscle (if normal) on the other side:
1. Use the unipolar technique (see Chap. 20) and continuous alternating current at 100 cycles per second.
2. Find the motor point of that muscle.
3. Slowly decrease/increase the intensity until an MPR is observed. The contraction should be barely visible.
4. Note and record the type of muscle response. The con-

traction should be rapid for a normal muscle.
5. Stimulate the muscle again. Read the meter and record the number milliamperes required to produce the MPR.
K. Repeat on the same muscle on the affected side:
   1. The minimal perceptible response must be of the same magnitude as that obtained from the corresponding muscle on the normal side.
L. If no response is obtained from the affected muscle with alternating current:
   1. Use interrupted direct current and repeat the entire procedure — normal and then abnormal muscle with the active electrode negative.
   2. Switch the current polarity and again find the MPR.
   3. Record the intensity and quality of the contraction.

## III. Terminating the Test

A. *Slowly* decrease the current intensity to zero or remove the active electrode during a break in the current.
B. Remove the electrodes.
C. Give the patient a dry turkish towel and tell (help) him to dry himself.
D. Turn off the unit and move it out of the patient's way.
E. Check the patient's skin. Remind him that it will be red for a little while and that the redness may come back if he takes a hot bath or shower.

## RHEOBASE AND CHRONAXIE

### Chronaxie Meter®: Teca Corporation

## I. Preparations

A. Determine the procedure to be used:
   1. Select the unit:
      a. The unit must either deliver direct current that can be interrupted manually or automatically by the

unit.
2. Select the technique:
    a. The unipolar technique is the technique of choice (see Chap. 20).
    b. The therapist should be skilled in electrical stimulation to assure accurate test results.
3. Select the electrodes:
    a. The active electrode should be small enough to stimulate the muscle being tested and to prevent current overflow as much as possible.
    b. The dispersive electrode should be at least 4 by 4 inches in size.
B. Have all materials ready to use:
    1. Wood plinth or table and chair.
    2. Warm water in which to soak the electrodes.
    3. Record form.
    4. Turkish towels.
C. Check the unit:
    1. Know how to operate the unit.
    2. All wire and plug connections should be tight.
    3. Do *not* use frayed conducting cords or electrode wires, corroded or loose-fitting wire tips, etc.
    4. Use wire tips that fit both the electrodes and the unit. Substitutions or makeshift connections can cause burns.
    5. Soak the electrodes in the warm water.
    6. Be sure the intensity control is off.
D. Type of muscle contraction. Use the minimal perceptible response, that response that is barely visible.

## II. Starting the Test

A. Explain the procedure to the patient:
    1. Describe the sensation he should feel. Use positive terms.
    2. He should know why the test is being done.
    3. Tell him that his skin may be red.
    4. *Demonstrate on yourself.* Get an actual contraction;

don't fake it.

    5. It may be necessary to let him feel the current on another part of his body before starting the test.

B.  Check the area to be tested:

    1. The skin should be clean and free from oils, lotions, and creams as these are insulators against electricity.

    2. Avoid stimulating on moles, new skin, recent scar tissue, cuts and abrasions.

C.  Check skin sensation. If sensation is lacking or diminished, use caution.

D.  *Never* stimulate *any* part of *any* patient who has an external or implanted electrical or atomic stimulating device such as a heart pacemaker.

E.  Do *not* stimulate:

    1. Directly over, through or in the vicinity of the heart.

    2. Any part of any patient who has a coronary problem.

    3. Directly through, over or near a recent or nonunion fracture site, the heart, or a pregnant uterus.

    4. Old scar tissue because it offers a great deal of resistance to current.

F.  Metal and electrical stimulation:

    1. Always use a wood plinth or table and chair.

    2. Remove (insulate) any metal in the area.

    3. Do *not* allow the patient to touch any metal while he is being treated.

G.  Reduce skin resistance by:

    1. Keeping the electrodes soaked throughout the test.

    2. Warming the cold skin with a superficial heat.

    3. Stimulating at least four times in the same place before moving the active electrode.

H.  Protect the sheet and patient's clothing from the water.

I.  Start on the *same* muscle on the normal side (if intact):

    1. Connect the active electrode to the negative pole.

    2. Set Pulse Duration, Duration Vernier and Intensity to zero.

    3. Set Duration Multiplier to X 1.

    4. Set Selector to RHEO.

    5. Set Interval to one second.

6. Set Output switch to on.
7. Find the motor point of the normal muscle and *stay on it throughout* the test. Moving the electrode will change the response.
8. *Slowly* increase/decrease the intensity until a minimal perceptible response is observed. The contraction should be barely visible.
9. Note and record the intensity required to produce the MPR. This intensity will be the *rheobase*.
10. Turn the Selector to CHRON.
11. Increase the Pulse Duration settings until an MPR is again observed.
12. Switch the Selector back to RHEO and recheck the rheobase.
13. If a minimal perceptible response is not observed, increase or decrease the intensity until one is seen.
14. Turn the Selector switch back to CHRON.
15. Readjust the Pulse Duration switch if necessary to again obtain the minimal perceptible response.
16. The minimal perceptible responses for both RHEO and CHRON must be *exactly* the same strength.
17. Record the Pulse Duration Dial settings.

J. Repeat the test on the suspect muscle on the affected side, and record the findings.

### III. Terminating the Test

A. Slowly decrease the intensity to zero.
B. Turn off the unit.
C. Remove the electrodes and have the patient dry himself.
D. Check the patient's skin.

### GALVANIC-TETANUS RATIO

### I. Preparations

A. Determine the procedure to be used:
   1. Select the unit:

a. The unit must either deliver direct current that can be interrupted manually or automatically by the unit.

2. Select the technique:
   a. The unipolar technique is the technique of choice. (see Chap. 20).
   b. The therapist should be skilled in electrical stimulation to assure accurate test results.

3. Select the electrodes:
   a. The active electrode should be small enough to stimulate the muscle being tested and to prevent current overflow as much as possible.

B. Have all materials ready to use:
   1. Wood plinth or table and chair.
   2. Warm water in which to soak the electrodes.
   3. Record form.
   4. Towels.

C. Check the unit:
   1. Know how to operate the unit.
   2. All wire and plug connections should be tight.
   3. Do *not* use frayed conducting cords or electrode wires, corroded or loose-fitting wire tips, etc.
   4. Use wire tips that fit both the electrodes and the unit. Substitutions or makeshift connections can cause burns.
   5. Soak the electrodes in the warm water.
   6. Be sure the intensity control is off.

## II. *Starting the Test*

A. Explain the procedure to the patient:
   1. Describe the sensation he should feel. Use positive terms.
   2. He should know why the test is being done.
   3. Tell him that his skin may be red.
   4. *Demonstrate on yourself.* Get an actual contraction; don't fake it.
   5. It may be necessary to let him feel the current on

another part of his body before starting the test.
B. Check the area to be tested:
　　1. The skin should be clean and free from oils, lotions, and creams as these are insulators against current.
　　2. Avoid stimulating on moles, new skin, recent scar tissue, cuts and abrasions.
C. Check skin sensation. If sensation is lacking or diminished, use caution.
D. *Never* stimulate *any* part of *any* patient who has an external or implanted electrical or atomic stimulating device such as a heart pacemaker.
E. Do *not* stimulate:
　　1. Directly over, through or in the vicinity of the heart.
　　2. Any part of any patient who has a coronary problem.
　　3. Directly through, over or near a recent or nonunion fracture site. the heart or a pregnant uterus.
　　4. Old scar tissue, because it offers a great deal of resistance to current.
F. Metal and electrical stimulation:
　　1. Always use a wood plinth or table and chair.
　　2. Remove (insulate) all metal in the area.
　　3. Do *not* allow the patient to touch any metal while he is being treated.
G. Reduce skin resistance by:
　　1. Keeping the electrodes soaked throughout the test.
　　2. Warming the cold skin with a superficial heat.
　　3. Stimulating at least four times in the same place before moving the active electrode.
H. Protect the sheet and patient's clothing from the water.
I. Start with the equivalent normal muscle (if intact) on the normal side:
　　1. Locate the motor point.
　　2. Find the minimal perceptible response.
　　3. Record the milliamperage required to produce the MPR.
　　4. Keep the active electrode on the motor point.
　　5. While making and breaking the current, advance the intensity rapidly until the muscle responds with a

tetanic contraction.

6. Record the milliamperage required to produce the tetanic contraction.
7. Divide the number of milliamperes required to produce the twitch (galvanic) response into the number of milliamperes required to produce the tetanic response.

J. Repeat the test on the same muscle on the affected side.
K. Record findings.

### III. Terminating the Test

A. Decrease the current intensity slowly.
B. Turn off the unit.
C. Remove the electrodes and have the patient dry himself.
D. Check the patient's skin.

*Chapter 22*

# TRANSCUTANEOUS ELECTRICAL NERVE STIMULATION

## *I. Preparations*

A. Determine the procedure to be used:
   1. Select the unit. There are many small, battery powered units available, or the standard department equipment may be used.

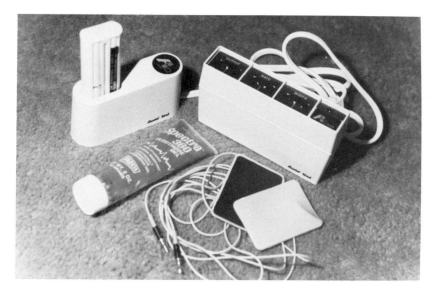

Figure 37. Transcutaneous electrical nerve stimulation unit and electrode gel. (Avery Corp. unit; Parker Laboratories gel)

   2. Type of current:
      A. Modulated direct current.
      b. Alternating current.
B. Check the unit to be used:

1. Battery powered units should be at full charge.
2. The line cord units should be grounded.
3. Know how to operate the unit.
4. Do *not* use frayed line cord or electrode wires, loose-fitting or corroded electrode tips, etc.
5. *Never* interchange electrodes or wires from unit to unit.
6. Use the correct wire tips. Substitutions or makeshift connections can cause burns.
7. Test the unit on yourself to be sure it is operating safely and efficiently.

C. Have all materials ready to use:
1. An electrode gel or lotion will be needed for battery powered units.
2. If padded electrodes or sponge inserts are used with large department units, soak them in warm water.
3. Gauze or cotton to cover padded electrodes and sponge inserts for hygienic purposes.
4. Turkish towels.

## II. Starting the Treatment

A. Do *not* stimulate:
1. *Any* part of *any* patient who has an implanted or external conventional or atomic stimulation device such as a cardiac pacemaker.
2. *Any* part of a patient with coronary heart disease.
3. In the area of or directly over or through the heart.
4. On recent scar tissue or new skin.
5. On open cuts or abrasions.
6. Directly on or near a recent or nonunion fracture site if the intensity is likely to cause a muscle contraction.

B. Explain the procedure to the patient:
1. Tell him why the treatment is being done.
2. Describe the sensation he should feel such as a prickly or tingly sensation or a muscle contraction.
3. Reassure him as many people are afraid of electricity.
4. Use positive terms. Do *not* say, "Don't be afraid," "You will be shocked," etc.

C. Demonstrate the treatment on yourself.

D. Allow the patient to feel the current on his forearm or on some area other than where the treatment will be.

E. Check the area to be treated:
   1. The skin should be clean and free from lotions, creams, oils, etc. as these are insulators against electricity.
   2. Check skin sensation. If sensation is lacking or diminished, use caution. Frequently during the first treatment, remove the electrodes and check the skin.
   3. Remove all metal in the area. All unremovable metal should be well padded with dry gauze or cotton and covered with plastic or rubber.

F. Any remaining clothing should be protected from water or electrode gels.

G. Prepare the electrodes:
   1. Padded electrodes or sponge inserts should be covered with gauze or cotton for hygienic purposes and then thoroughly soaked in warm water.
   2. When using rubber electrodes, check to be sure which side of the electrode conducts current. The conductive side must be covered with the conducting gel or lotion.

H. Attach the lead wires to the electrodes.

I. Warn the patient, and place the electrodes on his skin:
   1. Electrode placement is somewhat empirical. Five to ten patient visits may be necessary to determine which electrode placement produces the best results. They may be placed:
      a. On either side of the painful area.
      b. On the nerve roots at the spinal cord.
      c. On the peripheral nerves serving the painful area, and proximal or distal to the point of pain.
      d. On the painful area.
      e. On the nerve root and the painful area.
   2. Excellent and complete contact between the electrodes and the skin is essential throughout the treatment:
      a. The electrodes should not touch each other.
      b. Poor contact will result in an increased current density which can cause irritation.
      c. Hold the electrodes in place with the patient's body

weight, sandbags, straps, bandages, etc.

   3. *Always* turn the intensity control to zero *before* moving the electrode(s).

J. When using some battery powered units over a several month period and for several hours at a time, the current may produce polarity effects.

K. When skin irritation occurs, change the conducting medium if using a lotion or a gel, and/or change the position of the electrodes.

L. Attach the electrodes to the unit.

M. Check the unit to be sure the intensity (output/voltage) control is at zero.

N. Turn on the unit:

   1. Some battery powered units incorporate the on/off switch with the intensity control. If this is the case, turn on the unit *very slowly*.

O. When everything is ready, tell the patient you are going to turn on the current. Do *not* take him by surprise.

P. Adjust the stimulus. There is no one best setting. The optimum combination of settings for relief of pain can be obtained only by trial and error over a period of time for each patient. It may take from several minutes to several weeks to find the best combination:

   1. Intensity control:

      a. *Slowly* increase the intensity until the patient feels a prickly sensation or until a muscle contraction is obtained. (Usually TENS intensity is kept below that required to cause a muscle contraction.)

   2. Duration of the stimulus (width) and number of times the stimulus occurs (rate) are empirical:

      a. All changes in duration and rate settings should be done slowly.

      b. Some manufacturers recommend slowly decreasing the intensity to zero before varying the duration of the impulse.

Q. Treatment time:

   1. Allow at least two hours for the first treatment, depending on the patient's tolerance.

   2. After twenty minutes:

    a. Slowly turn the intensity to zero, remove the electrodes, and check the skin for any noxious reaction to the current or to the conducting medium.

    b. Ask the patient about any pain relief.

    c. Be sure he is comfortable and relaxed.

3. If the treatment time is three hours or more, check to be sure the gel has not dried out. If it has, remove the electrodes, wash the skin and electrodes and replace the gel. If you are using water, the electrodes may have to be resoaked after thirty minutes.

4. Total treatment time depends on:

    a. Each patient's tolerance to the current.

    b. The type of unit being used.

    c. The amount of pain relief. Some patients experience relief after a few minutes of stimulation. Others require from several hours to eight hours, and a few require continuous stimulation.

## III. *Terminating the Treatment*

A. *Slowly* turn the intensity control to zero.

B. Turn off the unit.

C. Remove the electrodes.

D. Give the patient a towel and tell (help) him to dry or wash his skin if gel has been used.

E. *Check the skin for any unusual marks that were not there before starting treatment.*

F. The patient's record should include:

    1. The dial settings for the intensity, width and rate.

    2. Exact electrode placement.

    3. Duration of the treatment.

    4. Amount of pain relief.

    5. Any untoward response.

    6. The specific unit used.

## IV. *Notes*

A. All electrodes should be washed or allowed to dry.

B.  Recharge batteries if using a battery powered unit.

## V. *Home Treatment*

A.  *Always* have the patient practice using the unit on himself in the department before he tries it at home.
B.  Instruct the patient:
    1.  How to remove and install batteries and how to charge the batteries.
    2.  How to use the electrodes:
        a.  Remind him that the intensity control should *always* be at zero *before* the electrodes are placed on his skin, removed and/or their position is changed.
        b.  Some electrodes are conductive on one side only.
        c.  The entire electrode surface should be covered with gel. If the electrodes are to be in place for three hours or longer, the gel should be checked for drying. If it has dried even slightly, the electrodes should be removed, electrodes and skin washed and the gel replaced.
        d.  Emphasize that complete and firm electrode contact is essential throughout the treatment.
C.  Tell the patient how long the treatment time should be and how often he should treat himself.
D.  Inform him of the precautions:
    1.  *Never* use or try the unit on *anyone* else including members of his own family, and tell him why.
    2.  Do *not* immerse the unit in any liquid.
    3.  Do *not* use near the eyes.
    4.  Keep out of reach of children.
    5.  Do not drop the unit.
    6.  Do not put the electrodes on open wounds.
    7.  Do not stimulate the throat or near the heart.
    8.  Do not use if pregnant.

*Chapter 23*

# MYOFEEDBACK

## *I. Preparations*

A. Determine the procedure to be used:
   1. Muscle reeducation.
   2. Muscle relaxation.
B. Select the electrodes:
   1. Invasive electrodes — needles, wires, etc.:
      a. Invasive electrodes are not recommended for rehabilitation procedures.
      b. These electrodes must be used for deep muscle and single motor unit pickup.
   2. Surface electrodes:
      a. These electrodes should be small (1 by 2.5 cm) so that the pickup will be as specific as possible.
      b. The electrodes may be square or circular metal plates with attached lead-off wires or suction cups.
      c. Some electrodes are flexible, and the spacing between them is fixed.
C. Select the electrode gel:
   1. An electrode gel must be used between the skin and the electrode to ensure complete contact of the electrode and to reduce the skin resistance as much as possible.
   2. A saline or powdered abrasive gel will effectively lower skin resistance.
   3. For long term use, nonsalt, hypoallergenic gels will be the least irritating to the skin.
D. Check the unit to be used:
   1. It is *mandatory* that line cord units be grounded:
      a. If a grounded outlet is not available, a three-prong to two-prong adapter may be used *temporarily* as long as the short wire from the adapter is long enough to be connected to a good electrical ground

such as a cold water pipe.
   b. Connect this wire *before* the power plug is connected.
   c. The power outlet should *not* have a branch circuit.
2. Be sure the battery powered units are at full charge.
3. Know how to operate the unit.
4. *Never* use defective equipment. The following are contraindications for treatment:
   a. Cracked insulation on power or connecting cables.
   b. Loose connections including electrode wires.
   c. Unusual heat, odors or sounds from the unit.
   d. Wet equipment whether wet from water or another liquid.
5. *Never connect a second power-line-operated unit to a patient who is attached to the myofeedback unit.*
6. Try the unit on yourself to be sure it is operating safely and efficiently.
E. A quiet room is helpful so the patient is able to hear when a muscle contracts or relaxes.
F. Interference:
   1. Potentials may be induced in the patient from any alternating current power lines:
      a. All treatment units, especially diathermy units, should not only be off, but unplugged and as far away from the myofeedback unit as possible.
      b. Any radio frequency energy such as that from hospital paging systems, television, police and taxi radios, etc. can be picked up by the unit.
      c. Ungrounded fluorescent lighting fixtures should be suspect.
      d. The examiner or observers can radiate 60 cycle interference. Touch the ground electrode or ground yourself by means of a ground wire if this is a problem.
G. Have all other necessary materials ready to use.

## II. Starting the Treatment

A. Metal:

1. *Never* put the patient on a metal plinth or chair or one that has metal parts.
2. *Never* allow the patient to come in contact with or touch any metal such as water pipes, electrical outlets or other operating units.

B. Patient's position:
1. The patient must be supported and as relaxed as possible.
2. The patient's position must allow you to work efficiently.

C. Explain the procedure to the patient:
1. He will not feel anything (unless invasive electrodes are used).
2. Select an unaffected muscle on the patient and demonstrate what he will hear and see. Have him listen and watch the visual display.
3. If an unaffected muscle is not easily available, demonstrate on yourself.
4. Give a goal to attain such as a specific number of microvolts on the meter or an increase/decrease in the auditory signal.

D. Check the area to be treated:
1. Remove all jewelry if appropriate.
2. The skin should be thoroughly washed.
3. Light abrading of the skin with gauze or sandpaper will remove dead skin and surface oils, which are insulators against current.

E. Electrode application:
1. Avoid scar tissue. It has a high electrical resistance that will decrease the strength of the signal.
2. Warn the patient.
3. Apply some electrode gel to the skin and to the electrodes:
   a. Too much gel may result in spreading of the gel between closely spaced electrodes, causing the electrodes to be short circuited.
   b. Spread the gel over the entire surface of the electrode.
   c. The skin between the two signal electrodes *must* be

clean and *dry*.
4. Signal (pick-up) electrodes:
   a. Place one of the signal electrodes on the motor point.
   b. Place the other electrode on the distal end of the same muscle belly or on the tendon of insertion.
   c. Avoid other muscles if possible.
   d. Straps or tape should be used to maintain excellent contact if the patient's body weight is not being used.
5. Patient ground electrode:
   a. Place the electrode at a point distant from the signal electrodes.
   b. Hold the electrode in place with the patient's body weight, tape or straps.
F. Muscle reeducation/facilitation:
   1. Initially, select a muscle with some voluntary control:
      a. If there are affected muscles on both the left and right sides of the body, select one on the patient's dominant side.
      b. Attach the electrodes.
      c. While he watches the *muscle,* have him contract it.
      d. Call his attention to the sound and to the visual display.
      e. Have him vary the amount of contraction, and point out the changes that occur in the sound produced and in the visual display.
   2. Attach the signal electrodes to a muscle with no apparent voluntary control:
      a. If intact, have the patient contract the same muscle on the *unaffected* side to get the "feel" of the contraction.
      b. Have the patient watch the muscle and listen as he attempts to contract the affected muscle.
      c. Use facilitation techniques if needed.
      d. When he can initiate a contraction, have him watch the visual display. Or if he cannot contract the muscle while looking at it, have him watch the meter/lights instead.

e. If the patient cannot elicit even a small contraction after repeated attempts, move to another muscle, and return to that first muscle later.

f. After a contraction can be repeated, give the patient auditory/visual goals to attain.

G. Muscle relaxation/inhibition:

1. Initially select an unaffected muscle:

a. Ask the patient to contract the muscle and hold the contraction.

b. Call his attention to both the sound and visual display.

c. Have him vary the amount of contraction, and point out the changes that occur in the sound produced and in the visual display.

d. Have him completely relax the muscle, and make him aware of the lack of any signal feedback.

e. Explain that silence and the lack of a visual display are the goals.

2. Attach the signal electrodes to the affected muscle:

a. Point out the high intensity of both the auditory and visual feedback.

b. Use relaxation techniques such as slow passive stretch if the muscle is spastic.

c. Ask the patient to concentrate on relaxing the muscle.

d. Have him stretch the muscle by contracting the antagonists on the unaffected side, and notice how it feels.

e. Repeat on the affected side.

f. When any relaxation is accomplished, point out the decreases in audio and visual activity.

H. Treatment time:

1. Treatment time will vary according to the patient's tolerance.

2. If the patient becomes frustrated or tired, discontinue treatment.

3. The amount of voluntary muscle control and/or the number of muscles to be treated will also determine the

treatment time.

## III. *Terminating the Treatment*

A. Turn off the unit.
B. Remove the electrodes.
C. Give the patient a towel and tell (help) him to wipe his skin.
D. Check the patient's skin.
E. Record the number of microvolts attained and an increase/decrease of the auditory signal.
F. A graphic representation can motivate the patient.
G. Clean the electrodes.

# Part VI
# Ultraviolet Techniques

*Chapter 24*

# MINIMAL ERYTHEMAL DOSE TEST

## Local Cold Quartz Lamp

### *I. Preparations*

A.  Determine the procedure to be used:
   1. Do the test on a part of the body where the skin color is the *same* as the area to be treated.
   2. If you will treat skin of different shades, more than one MED test will be required.

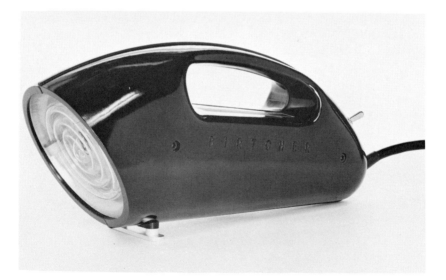

Figure 38. Local Spot quartz ultraviolet lamp. (Courtesy of Birtcher Corp.)

B.  Check the lamp:
   1. Know how to operate the lamp.

197

   2. The quartz tube should be clean:
      a. Use Bon Ami, distilled water or absolute alcohol. Do *not* use rubbing alcohol.
      b. Do *not* touch the tube as perspiration can damage it.
C. If the lamp has not been used for some time, find your own MED several days before the patient is to be tested. This can help you determine the approximate exposure time to use to start the patient's test.
D. Practice handling the lamp.
E. Lamp warm-up time is thirty seconds.
F. Use a towel to shield the radiation. Do *not* cover any air vents.
G. Have all materials ready to use:
   1. Goggles. Regular eyeglasses or dark glasses are *not* acceptable. They will shut out the harmful radiation that comes directly at them; however, radiation can come in around the edges of glasses.
   2. Watch. A watch with a second hand is *mandatory*. A timer is not acceptable because of the short times used.
   3. Cut out paper towel or card:
      a. Take a paper towel and cut out or tear out four holes 1/2 inch in diameter or less, side by side, in a row. Leave approximately 1 inch of space between each cutout to allow for draping.
   4. Drape sheet, towels, etc.

## II. Starting the Test

A. Explain the procedure to the patient:
   1. He should know why the test is being done.
   2. Tell him that he should get a sunburn, and that it will occur in four small places.
   3. Explain why the test takes such a short time.
   4. Tell him his eyes must be protected as well as all other skin not being tested, and tell him why.
   5. If you use the word *radiation*, reassure the patient that this is not like atomic radiation.

B. The therapist should stay out of the radiation as much as possible.

C. Position the patient so he will be comfortable throughout the test:
   1. The volar surface of the forearm may be used for the test.
   2. Use pillows for comfort and support.

D. Drape the patient:
   1. Proper and complete draping is essential.
   2. All skin areas, including the head, that are not being tested *must* be draped.
   3. The head may be left uncovered until the test begins.

E. The skin should be clean and free from oils, lotions and creams.

F. Do *not* test on:
   1. New skin.
   2. Scar tissue.
   3. Sunburn.
   4. Skin rash, abrasions, cuts.
   5. Skin hair. If the hair on the skin is thick, use another area if possible. If not possible, then with the patient's permission, the hair should be shaved.

G. Ask the patient to put on goggles:
   1. If the patient's head will be completely covered and the draping is secure, goggles are not necessary. But if available, they should be used.
   2. Warn the patient never to look at the radiation even with goggles on and tell him why.
   3. Children, the elderly, developmentally delayed and psychotic patients demand special attention.

H. Place the test guide on the skin to be tested. Use a skin pencil and place a dot on the skin next to each cutout. Remind the patient not to wash off the dots for at least twelve hours after the test.

I. Use the drape sheet or a towel to hold the guide in place and to cover all exposed areas around the guide.

J. Cover the cutouts with a hand or turkish towel.

K. Place another towel lengthwise at one end of the row of

cutouts.
L.  *Put goggles on yourself:*
   1.  Ultraviolet should *never* be given unless goggles are available for the therapist (and anyone in the treatment booth). Do *not* use regular eyeglasses or dark glasses as substitutes as radiation can come in around the edges of the glasses.
   2.  If only one pair of goggles is available, *you* wear them, and make certain the patient's eyes are protected.
   3.  *Never* look directly at the ultraviolet source even with goggles on.
M.  Be *sure* you can read the seconds or second hand on a watch *before* you start timing:
   1.  Goggles may be worn under glasses, but not over them unless the goggles completely enclose the glasses.
   2.  If you cannot see the seconds or second hand, *never* estimate the time. Have another staff person time for you from outside the booth unless goggles are available for him.
N.  Tell the patient you are about to start the test and that he should not move, and tell him why.
O.  The distance from the lamp to the exposed skin can be from contact to 1 inch:
   1.  One inch is recommended for hygienic reasons.
   2.  Keep the spacing uniform for each exposure.
P.  The lamp *must* be held at a *right angle* to the skin.
Q.  Turn on the lamp and cover the tube with a towel.
R.  The exposure time sequence will vary:
   1.  The color of the patient's skin and the number of hours the lamp has been used will determine the initial exposure time.
   2.  At a spacing of 1 inch on white skin using a new lamp, a minimal erythemal dose should be obtained at six seconds.
   3.  Two, four, six, and eight second sequence may be used on white skin. Albinos and redheads may need to have one, two, three, and four seconds.
S.  Drape the patient's head, and recheck other draping.

T.  Keeping all cutouts covered, hold the lamp in your dominant hand, remove the towel, and rest the lamp on its face on the plinth.

U.  Expose as follows (at 1 inch of spacing and at a right angle):
1.  With your nondominant hand, uncover the first cutout. Expose the skin for *two seconds*; place the lamp on its face on the plinth; cover the tested cutout with the drape towel at the end of the row of cutouts.
2.  Using the same technique, uncover the second cutout; expose it for *four seconds*; cover the cutout.
3.  Uncover the third cutout; expose it for *six seconds*.
4.  Uncover the fourth cutout; expose it for *eight seconds*.

## III. Terminating the Treatment

A.  Turn off the lamp. (There is no need to leave the lamp on if another patient is to follow.)
B.  Rehang the lamp or put it under the plinth out of the patient's way, and remove the draping and goggles.
C.  *Tell the patient:*
1.  *What* to look for:
    a.  He should look for the cutout showing the *lightest* pink color.
    b.  The exposure time for that lightest pink color will be *that* patient's MED for *that* lamp.
    c.  He may see nothing or he may see all red spots.
2.  *Where* to look for the lightest pink color:
    a.  The patient must know which cutout was exposed for the longest (shortest) time.
    b.  Tell him to write down which cutout showed the lightest pink color as you must know before you can treat him.
3.  *When* to look:
    a.  The patient should start checking the tested area in from three to four hours.
    b.  It may take up to twelve hours. Remind him again not to wash off the pencil dots for twelve hours.

     c. The color on the skin exposed for the *longest* time will appear first.

D.  If there was no reaction:
1. Repeat the test on another area.
2. The spacing between the lamp and skin may have been too great.
3. The lamp may not have been held at a right angle.
4. The exposure times may not have been long enough.

E.  If only red areas appeared:
1. Repeat the test on another area of the body.
2. Reduce the exposure times for each cutout.

F.  The patient's record should include:
1. Date of the test.
2. On what specific body area the test was done.
3. The exposure times used for each cutout.
4. Which cutout was exposed for the least/most amount of time.
5. The specific lamp used:
    a. If there are two or more local cold quartz lamps in your department, you must use the *same* lamp to treat the patient as you used for his test.
    b. Identify the lamp by the serial number, color, etc.

H.  The patient's MED should be rechecked:
1. At least every six months.
2. If the skin to be treated has changed color (tanned) since his last treatment.
3. If he is now getting drugs such as sulfa, quinine, or the tetracyclene group; endocrines such as insulin or thyroxin; heavy metals such as gold.

## LOCAL HOT QUARTZ LAMP

### *I. Preparations*

A.  Determine the procedure to be used:
1. Do the test on a part of the body where the skin color is the *same* as the skin to be treated.
2. If you will treat skin of different shades, more than one

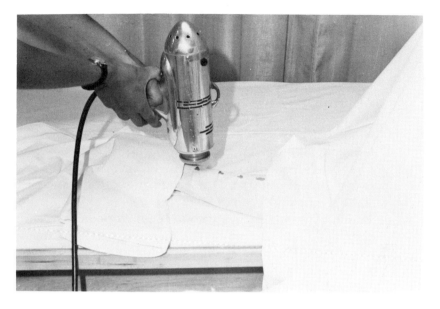

Figure 39. Local hot quartz lamp; MED test.

test will be required.
B. Check the lamp:
  1. Know how to operate the lamp.
  2. The lens should be clean:
     a. Be sure to clean the lens and not the lens filter.
     b. Do *not* touch the lens with your fingers as perspiration can damage it.
     c. Use Bon Ami, distilled water or absolute alcohol. Do *not* use rubbing alcohol.
  3. The filter should be in place over the lens:
     a. If the filter is missing, a towel should be used over the lens to prevent the escape of radiation.
     b. The towel must *not* cover any air vents.
C. If the lamp has not been used for some time, find your own MED several days before the patient is to be tested. This can help you determine the approximate exposure time to use to start the patient's test. (Be sure to use the same lamp on the patient.)
D. Practice handling the lamp, as it is awkward and heavy.

E. Warm up the lamp *before* the patient comes in:
1. The lens should be covered and pointed away from the treatment area.
2. Turn on the lamp.
3. Do *not* use the lamp if the fan is not operating.
4. The warm-up time is five to ten minutes depending on the number of hours the tube has been used.
F. Have all materials ready to use:
1. Goggles. Regular eyeglasses or dark glasses are *not* acceptable. They will shut out the harmful radiation that comes directly at them; however, radiation can reach the eyes around the edges of the lenses.
2. Watch. A watch with a second hand or one that clearly shows the seconds, while the therapist's hand is free to handle the lamp, is *mandatory*. A timer is not acceptable due to the short times used.
3. Spacers. If available, they should be used to assure uniform spacing between the lens and the skin.
4. Test guide. Take a paper towel or card and cut out or tear out four holes 1/2 inch in diameter or less, side by side in a row. Leave approximately 1 inch of space between each cutout to allow for draping.
5. Drape sheet, towels, etc.

## II. Starting the Test

A. Explain the procedure to the patient:
1. He should know why the test is being done.
2. Tell him that he should get a sunburn and that it will occur in four small areas.
3. Explain why the test takes such a short time.
4. Tell him his eyes must be protected as well as all other skin not being treated, and tell him why.
B. The therapist should stay out of the radiation as much as possible.
C. Position the patient so he will be comfortable throughout the test:
1. The volar surface of the forearm may be used for the

test.
2. Use pillows for comfort and support.
D.  Drape the patient:
    1. Proper and complete draping is essential.
    2. All skin areas, including the head, that are not being tested *must* be draped.
    3. The head may be left uncovered until the test begins.
E.  The skin should be clean and free from oils, lotions and creams.
F.  Do *not* test on:
    1. New skin.
    2. Scar tissue.
    3. Sunburn.
    4. Skin rash, abrasion, etc.
    5. Skin hair. If the hair on the skin is thick, use another area ,if possible. If not, then with the patient's permission, the hair should be shaved.
G.  Ask the patient to put on goggles:
    1. If the patient's head will be completely covered and the draping is secure, goggles are not necessary. But if available, they should be used.
    2. Warn the patient never to look at the radiation even with goggles on, and tell him why.
    3. Children, the elderly, retarded and psychotic patients demand special attention.
H.  Place the test guide on the skin to be tested. Use a skin pencil and place a dot on the skin next to each cutout. Remind the patient not to wash off the dots for at least twelve hours after the test.
I.  Use the drape sheet or a towel to hold the guide in place and to cover all exposed areas around the guide.
J.  *Put goggles on yourself:*
    1. Ultraviolet should *never* be given unless goggles are available for the therapist (and anyone in the treatment booth). Do *not* use regular eyeglasses or dark glasses as substitutes as radiation can come in around the edges of the lenses.
    2. If only one pair of goggles is available, *you* wear them,

and make certain the patient's eyes are protected.

3. *Never* look directly at the ultraviolet source even with goggles on.

K. Be *sure* you can read the seconds or second hand on your watch *before* you start timing:

1. Goggles may be worn under glasses but not over them unless the goggles completely enclose the glasses.

2. If you cannot see the seconds, *never* estimate the time. Have another staff person time for you from outside of the treatment booth (unless goggles are available for him).

L. Tell the patient you are about to start the test and that he should not move, and tell him why.

M. Either unhook the warmed-up lamp from the snap hook or leaving it attached, pull it down to the test area.

N. The distance from the lens to the exposed skin is usually from 1 to 1 1/2 inches:

1. Use spacers if available.

2. Keep the spacing uniform for each exposure.

O. The lamp *must* be held at a *right angle* to the skin.

P. The exposure time sequence may vary:

1. Four, eight, twelve and sixteen seconds are the usual exposure times.

2. Albinos and redheads may require two, four, six and eight seconds.

3. The longer the lamp has been used, the longer the exposure must be to produce an MED.

Q. Drape the patient's head, and recheck the other draping.

R. Keeping all cutouts covered, hold the lamp in your dominant hand over the plinth, remove the towel or filter and let the lamp rest on the lens on the plinth. Do not put the lamp down on the plinth as the housing will be very hot and a fire could result.

S. Expose as follows:

1. With your nondominant hand, uncover the first cutout; expose the skin for *four seconds*; rest the lamp on its lens on the plinth; cover the cutout with the towel.

2. Uncover the second cutout; expose it for *eight seconds*;

place the lamp on its lens; cover the tested area.
3. Uncover the third cutout; expose it for *twelve seconds*; etc.
4. Uncover the fourth cutout; expose it for *sixteen seconds;* cover immediately.

## III. Terminating the Treatment

A. Replace the lens filter or towel. Do *not* cover the air vents.
B. Retract or rehang the lamp.
C. Turn off the lamp and move it back out of the patient's way. (If another patient is to be tested/treated within twenty minutes, leave the lamp on to avoid the necessary cooling and reheating times.)
D. Remove the patient's goggles.
E. *Tell the patient:*
   1. *What* to look for:
      a. He should look for the cutout showing the lightest pink color. (The exposure time for the lightest pink color will be *that* patient's MED for *that* lamp.)
      b. He may see nothing or he may see only red areas.
   2. *Where* to look for the lightest pink color:
      a. He must know which cutout was exposed for the least/most amount of time.
      b. Warn the patient again about washing off the dots before twelve hours.
   3. *When* to look:
      a. The patient should start checking the area in three to four hours.
      b. It may take up to twelve hours for the lightest pink color to appear.
      c. The color on the skin exposed for the longest time will appear first.
   4. He must remember where the MED appeared as you must know before he can be treated.
F. If there was no reaction:
   1. Repeat the test several days before treating the patient.
   2. The distance between the lens and skin might have

been too much.
   3. The lamp may not have been held at a right angle.
   4. The lamp may not have had sufficient preheating time.
   5. The exposure times may have been too short.
G. If only red areas appeared:
   1. Repeat the test on another area of the body.
   2. Reduce the exposure times for each cutout.
H. The patient's record should include:
   1. Date of the test.
   2. The specific body area on which the test was done.
   3. The exposure time for each cutout.
   4. Which cutout was exposed for the least/most amount of time.
   5. Specific lamp used:
      a. If there are two or more local hot quartz lamps in your department, you must use the *same* lamp to treat that patient as you used to find his MED.
      b. Identify the lamp by the serial number, color, etc.
I. The patient's MED should be rechecked:
   1. At least every six months.
   2. If the skin to be treated has changed color (tanned) since his last treatment.
   3. If he is now getting drugs such as sulfa, quinine, or the tetracyclene group; endocrines such as insulin or thyroxin; heavy metals such as gold.

**GENERAL HOT QUARTZ LAMP**

*I. Preparations*

A. Determine the procedure to be used:
   1. Do the test on a part of the body where the skin color is the *same* as the skin on the area to be treated.
   2. If you will treat skin of different shades, more than one MED test will be required.
B. Check the lamp:
   1. Know how to operate the lamp and the adjustments *before* the patient comes in for the test.

2. Do *not* use the lamp if the shutters are not working properly.
3. The quartz tube, lamp hood and shutter reflectors should be clean and dust free:
   a. Do *not* touch the quartz tube as perspiration can damage it.
   b. Use Bon Ami, distilled water or absolute alcohol. Do *not* use rubbing alcohol.
4. Know where the quartz tube is attached to the hood as this reference point is used for measuring the distance between the source of the radiation and the skin.
5. If the lamp has not been used for some time, find your MED several days before the patient is to be tested. This can help you determine the approximate exposure time to use to start the patient's test. (Be sure to use the same lamp on the patient.)

D. Warm up the lamp *before* the patient comes in:
   1. Be *sure* the shutters are tightly closed.
   2. If using a combination ultraviolet/infrared lamp, turn on the correct switch.
   3. The warm-up time is usually five to ten minutes depending on the number of hours the tube has been used.
   4. The shutters *must* remain tightly closed during the warm-up time and until timing actually begins.
   5. *Never* cover the lamp hood as it will get hot and a fire may result. (Some radiation will inevitably escape between the cracks of the shutters.)

E. Have all materials ready to use:
   1. Goggles. Regular eyeglasses or dark glasses are *not* acceptable. They will shut out the harmful radiation that comes directly at them; however, radiation can reach the eyes by coming in around the edges of the lenses.
   2. Watch. A watch with a second hand or one that clearly shows the seconds while the therapist's hand is free to move the draping is *mandatory*. A timer may be used, but timing is more accurate with a second hand.
   3. Tape measure:

    a. *Never* estimate the spacing. A tape measure is *mandatory* to measure the *exact* distance between the *source* of the ultraviolet and the highest area to be treated.

    b. A steel tape measure or one made of unstretchable material is preferable.

    c. Some lamps have a tape measure built into the lamp on the outside of the hood at the level of the quartz tube.

  4. Test guide:

    a. Take a paper towel or card and cut out or tear out four holes 1/2 inch in diameter or less, side by side in a row. Leave approximately 1 inch of space between each cutout to allow for draping.

  5. Two drape sheets, towels, etc.

## II. Starting the Test

A. Explain the procedure to the patient:
  1. He should know why the test is being done.
  2. Tell him that he should get a sunburn, but that it occurs in four small areas.
  3. Explain why the test takes such a short time.
  4. Tell him his eyes must be protected as well as all other skin not being tested, and tell him why.
  5. If you use the word *radiation,* assure the patient that it is not the same as atomic radiation.

B. The therapist should stay out of the radiation as much as possible.

C. Position the patient so he will be comfortable throughout the treatment:
  1. Use the abdomen for the test.
  2. Place the patient supine on the plinth with a pillow under his head and one under his knees.

D. Drape the patient:
  1. Proper and complete draping is essential.
  2. Place one drape sheet over the upper half of the body, leaving the head uncovered until the lamp is brought

over the patient.

   3. Drape the lower half of the patient with another sheet, but leave the abdomen exposed.

E. The skin on the abdomen should be clean and free from oils, lotions, creams, etc.:

   1. Do *not* test on scar tissue or new skin.

   2. Do *not* test on sunburn.

   3. If the skin hair is thick, it should be shaved (with permission of the patient), or another area may be used.

F. Ask the patient to put on goggles:

   1. If the patient's head will be completely covered and the draping is secure, goggles are not necessary. But if available, they should be used.

   2. Warn the patient never to look at the radiation even with the goggles on, and tell him why.

   3. Children, the elderly, psychotic and retarded patients will require special attention.

G. Tell the patient what you are going to do, and place the test guide on the abdomen above the navel so the cutouts run across the exposed area.

H. Using a skin pencil, place a dot *next* to each area to be tested.

I. Drape any exposed areas around the test guide with the drape sheet and/or towels.

J. Cover the cutouts with a hand towel or turkish towel.

K. Cover the patient's head. Be sure he can breathe properly.

L. Move the lamp over the patient.

M. Measure thirty inches *perpendicularly* from the *source* of the ultraviolet to the skin highest to the source:

   1. Use the lamp adjustments.

   2. The measurement may be taken from *outside* the hood where the ultraviolet tube attaches to the hood, or the spacing may be measured from the bottom edge of the lamp (not the shutter) to the skin, providing compensation has been made for the distance between that edge and the tube. (Do *not* touch the tube.)

   3. Measurement and angle should be exact.

N. Center the lamp lengthwise and crosswise over the abdomen.
O. Adjust the hood so the radiation will be at a *right* angle to the abdomen.
P. *Put goggles on yourself.*
   1. Ultraviolet should *never* be given unless goggles are available for the therapist. Do *not* use regular eyeglasses or dark glass as substitutes for goggles.
   2. If only one pair of goggles is available, *you* wear them, and make sure the patient's eyes are covered.
   3. *Never* look at the ultraviolet source even with goggles on.
Q. Be *sure* you can read the seconds or second hand on your watch *before* starting to time:
   1. Goggles may be worn under eyeglasses but not over them unless the goggles completely enclose the glasses.
   2. If you cannot see the seconds on your watch, *never* estimate the time. Have another staff person time for you from outside of the booth (unless goggles are available for him).
R. Tell the patient that you are about to start the test and that he should not move, and tell him why.
S. Remove the cutout draping, but leave the towel at one end of the test guide.
T. Open the shutters wide enough to allow the radiation to reach all cutouts.
U. Start timing *immediately:*
   1. At the end of fifteen seconds, cover the first cutout. (Do *not* close the shutters.)
   2. At the end of an additional fifteen seconds (total of thirty seconds), cover the second cutout.
   3. At the end of another fifteen seconds (total of forty-five seconds), cover the third cutout.
   4. At the end of sixty seconds, either cover, or close the shutters.
V. An alternate method is to leave all cutouts covered and progressively uncover them.

### III. Terminating the Test

A. If another patient is to be tested within twenty minutes, leave the lamp on to avoid the necessary cooling and re-heating time. If the lamp is turned off, open the shutters to allow faster cooling. Some lamps cannot be restarted until they have cooled.

B. Turn off the lamp. Move it to the back of the booth out of the patient's way.

C. Remove the patient's goggles.

D. *Tell the patient:*
  1. *What* to look for:
     a. He should look for the cutout showing the lightest pink color. (The exposure time for the cutout showing the lightest pink color will be that patient's MED for *that* lamp.)
     b. He may see nothing or he may see only red spots.
  2. *Where* to look:
     a. The patient must know which cutout was exposed for the least/most amount of time.
     b. Warn the patient about washing off the dots for at least twelve hours.
  3. *When* to look:
     a. The patient should start checking the area in three to four hours.
     b. It may take up to twelve hours for the lightest pink color to appear.
     c. The color on the skin exposed for the longest time will appear first.

E. Tell the patient to write down which cutout showed the lightest pink color as you must know this before you can treat him.

F. Warn the patient not to touch the lamp hood as it will be hot.

G. If there was no reaction:
  1. The test *must* be repeated several days before treatment can be given.

    2. The lamp may not have had sufficient warm-up time.

    3. The exposure times might have been too short.

H.  If only red areas appear, repeat the test on another part of the body and reduce the exposure times.

I.   The patient's record should include:

    1. The date of the test.

    2. The *specific* body area on which the test was done.

    3. The exposure time for each cutout.

    4. Which cutout was exposed for the least/most amount of time.

    5. Specific lamp used:

        a. If there are two or more general lamps in your department, you must use the *same* lamp to treat that patient as you used to find his MED.

        b. Identity the lamp by the serial number, color, etc.

J.  The patient's MED should be rechecked:

    1. At least every six months.

    2. If the skin to be treated has changed color (tanned) since his last treatment.

    3. If he is now getting drugs such as sulfa, quinine, or the tetracyclene group; endocrines such as insulin or thyroxin; heavy metals such as gold.

*Chapter 25*

# ULTRAVIOLET GENERAL EXPOSURE

## *I. Preparations*

A. Determine the procedure to be used:
    1. Select the patient's position.
    2. The patient's minimal erythemal dose time *must* be known. If you will treat areas of different skin colors, MED's will have to be done for each area. The patient's MED should be rechecked:
        a. At least every six months.
        b. If the skin to be treated has changed color since the patient's last treatment.
        c. If the patient is now getting drugs such as sulfa, quinine, or the tetracyclene group; endocrines such as insulin or thyroxin; heavy metals such as gold.
B. Select the lamp:
    1. The lamp must be the *same* lamp that was used to determine that patient's MED.
    2. The same kind of lamp made by the same manufacturer *cannot* be used as the hour age of the tube may be different from that of the lamp used to test the patient.
C. Check the lamp:
    1. Know how to operate the lamp and lamp adjustments *before* the patient comes in for treatment.
    2. Do *not* use the lamp if the shutters are not working properly.
    3. The quartz tube, hood and shutter reflectors should be clean and dust free:
        a. Do *not* touch the tube as perspiration can damage it.
        b. Use Bon Ami, distilled water or absolute alcohol to clean the tube and reflectors. Do *not* use rubbing alcohol.

215

4. Know where the quartz tube is attached to the hood, as this reference point is used for measuring the distance between the source of the radiation and the skin.

C. Warm up the lamp *before* the patient comes in:
   1. The shutters *must* remain tightly closed during the warm-up time and until timing actually begins.
   2. If using a combination ultraviolet/infrared lamp, turn on the correct switch.
   3. The warm-up time is usually five to ten minutes, depending on the number of hours the tube has been used.
   4. *Never* cover the lamp hood as it will get hot and a fire may result. Some radiation will inevitably escape from between the cracks of the shutters.

D. Have all materials ready to use:
   1. Goggles. Regular eyeglasses or dark glasses are *not* acceptable. They will shut out the harmful radiation that comes directly at them; however, radiation can reach the eyes by coming in around the edges of the lenses.
   2. Watch. A watch with a second hand or one that clearly shows the seconds, or a timer is *mandatory*.
   3. Tape measure:
      a. *Never* estimate the spacing. A tape measure is *mandatory* to measure the *exact* distance between the *source* of the ultraviolet and the highest area to be treated.
      b. A steel tape measure or one made of unstretchable material is preferable.
      c. Some lamps have a tape measure built into the lamp on the outside of the hood at the level of the quartz tube.
   4. Two drape sheets will be needed.

E. Exposure times for each area (if the sunburn from the previous treatment has subsided and if the patient is treated every other day):
   1. First treatment. Use the patient's MED time.
   2. Second treatment. Double the MED time, or the MED time may be increased by fifteen seconds.
   3. Third treatment. Triple the MED time or the MED

time may be increased by thirty seconds.

4. When a weekend intervenes, use the same exposure time that was used on the previous Friday.
5. If one week or more passes between treatments, use the originial MED time when resuming treatments.

## II. Starting the Treatment

A. When exposing the entire body to ultraviolet:
   1. Use four exposures on an adult — upper half of the body and then the lower half when the patient is supine (prone) and then repeat on the other side.
   2. A child may be treated with one exposure on each side.
B. Explain the procedure to the patient:
   1. Tell him he should get a mild sunburn.
   2. Explain why the treatment takes such a short time.
   3. Tell him his eyes must be protected as well as all other skin not being treated, and tell him why.
   4. If you use the word *radiation,* reassure the patient that ultraviolet is not the same as atomic radiation.
C. The therapist should stay out of the radiation as much as possible.
D. Have the patient completely undress, and provide him with a T-binder or other appropriate clothing:
   1. Provide women with a large turkish towel folded lengthwise to cover the breasts.
   2. If the genital or breast areas must be treated, see General Exposure to the Undraped Patient.
E. Tell the patient to get onto the table, lie on his back and cover himself with the drape sheet:
   1. *Put his arms in the reverse T position:*
     a. The upper extremities may be placed in any position. However, to avoid a double exposure, they must be in the *same* position when the patient is prone.
   2. The patient will probably be more comfortable with a pillow under his head.
   3. He should have a pillow under his knees.
F. The skin should be clean and free from oils, creams and

lotions:
1. Cover all new skin and recent scar tissue.
2. Do *not* treat sunburned skin.
3. If the skin hair is thick, it may have to be shaved.
G. Cover the patient's eyes with thick, wet gauze or cotton pads:
    1. When treating the face, do *not* have the patient wear goggles.
    2. Tell the patient to keep his eyes closed and not to move.
H. Cover the patient's head with the drape sheet:
    1. The patient's face should be covered until immediately before timing begins to prevent exposure to the radiation coming from where the shutters meet.
    2. Be sure the patient can breathe easily.
I. Move the lamp over the upper (lower) half of the patient:
    1. Tell the patient what you are doing.
    2. Measure *exactly* 30 inches from the source of the ultraviolet to the skin nearest to the tube:
        a. Take the measurement from the *outside* of the hood where the ultraviolet tube attaches (to avoid touching the tube) or
        b. You may measure from the bottom of the lamp hood to the highest area to be treated, but be sure to allow for the extra distance from the edge of the hood to the tube.
        c. Loosen the correct lamp adjustments *before* raising or lowering the lamp.
    3. Center the lamp lengthwise and crosswise over the upper half (lower half) of the body including the head.
    4. Use the hood adjustments and move the hood so the radiation will be at a *right angle* to the skin.
J. *Put goggles on yourself:*
    1. Ultraviolet should *never* be given unless goggles are available for the therapist. Do *not* use regular eyeglasses or dark glasses as substitutes for goggles.
    2. If only one pair of goggles is available, *you* wear them, and make certain the patient's eyes are covered.

3. *Never* look directly at the ultraviolet source even with goggles on.

K. Be *sure* you can read the seconds or second hand on your watch *before* you start timing:

　　1. Goggles may be worn under glasses but not over them unless the goggles completely enclose the glasses.

　　2. If you cannot see the seconds on your watch, *never* estimate the time. Have another staff person time for you from outside of the booth (unless goggles are available for him).

　　3. An interval timer may be used.

L. With the patient holding his draping in place, fold down the top (bottom) half of the drape sheet:

　　1. If folding down the upper half of the drape sheet, be sure to tell the patient to keep his eyes closed.

　　2. The upper (bottom) edge of the umbilicus or the anterior superior iliac spines should be used as markers for the end of the drape sheet.

　　3. Recheck to be sure all areas that are not going to be exposed are properly draped.

M. Check the position of the upper extremities so this *same* position will be used when the patient is prone.

N. Open the shutters only wide enough to allow the radiation to reach to the sides of the body. Use the shutter knobs as the shutters will be very hot.

O. Start timing immediately.

P. Close the shutters *exactly* on time.

Q. Redrape the upper half of the patient including his head.

R. Move the lamp over the lower half of the body.

S. Remove the pillow from under the knees and place it under the head (if the patient does not already have one).

T. Measure 30 inches from the source of ultraviolet to the highest point to be treated.

U. Center the lamp lengthwise and crosswise.

V. Tell the patient to hold onto his draping, and pull up the lower half of the drape sheet:

　　1. Use the *same* markers for the bottom half of the drape sheet as you used for the first exposure. This is impor-

tant in order to avoid a double exposure at the waist.
   2. If the patient has his upper extremities at his sides, be sure his wrists and hands are draped.
W. Expose the lower half of the body for the same length of time as was used on the upper half.
X. Redrape the patient.
Y. Turn the patient to the prone position:
   1. Place the head pillow under the abdomen.
   2. Measure, center the lamp and expose as you did on the anterior surface of the patient.

## III. Terminating the Treatment

A. If another patient is to follow within twenty minutes, leave the lamp on to avoid the necessary cooling and reheating time. If the lamp is turned off, open the shutters to allow faster cooling. Some lamps cannot be restarted until they have cooled.
B. Turn off the lamp, and move it to the back of the treatment booth out of the patient's way.
C. Remove the patient's goggles.
D. Tell the patient:
   1. He can expect a mild sunburn.
   2. It should appear in from six to twelve hours.
E. The patient's record should include:
   1. Date of the treatment.
   2. The exposure time used.
   3. The distance from the source to the patient.
   4. Specific lamp used. Identify the lamp by the serial number, color, etc.

*Chapter 26*

# GENERAL EXPOSURE TO THE UNDRAPED PATIENT

## *I. Preparations*

A. Determine the procedure to be used:
   1. This procedure should be practiced several times with the lamp off before the patient is treated.
   2. If at all possible, the therapist should remain outside of the treatment booth any time the breast and/or genital areas of an adult are to be treated.
   3. From the age of five or six years, children should be treated by a therapist of the same sex.
   4. Age, puberty, religious objections, etc. should determine the selection of this method of treatment.
B. Select the lamp:
   1. The lamp must be the *same* one that was used to determine that patient's MED.
   2. The same kind of lamp made by the same manufacturer *cannot* be used as the hour age of the tube may be different from that of the lamp used to test the patient.
C. The patient's minimal erythemal dose time *must* be known. If you will treat areas of different skin colors, MED's will have to be done for each area. The patient's MED should be rechecked:
   1. At least every six months.
   2. If the skin to be treated has changed color since the patient's last treatment.
   3. If the patient is now getting drugs such as sulfa, quinine, or the tetracyclene group; endocrines such as insulin or thyroxin; heavy metals such as gold.
D. Check the lamp:
   1. Know how to operate the lamp and the adjustments *before* the patient comes in.

2. Do *not* use the lamp if the shutters are not working properly.
3. The quartz tube and hood and shutter reflectors should be clean and dust free:
   a. Do *not* touch the tube with your fingers, as perspiration may damage it.
   b. Use Bon Ami, distilled water, or absolute alcohol. Do *not* use rubbing alcohol.
4. Know where the quartz tube is attached to the hood as this reference point is used for measuring the distance between the source of the radiation and the skin.

E. Warm up the lamp *before* the patient comes in:
   1. The shutters *must* remain tightly closed during the warm-up period and until timing actually begins.
   2. If using a combination ultraviolet/infrared lamp, turn on the correct switch.
   3. The warm-up time is usually five to ten minutes depending on the number of hours the tube has been used.
   4. *Never* cover the lamp hood as it will get hot and a fire may result. (Some radiation will inevitably escape from between the shutters.)

F. Have all materials ready to use:
   1. Goggles. Regular eyeglasses or dark glasses are *not* acceptable. They will shut out the harmful radiation coming directly at them, but they cannot shut out the radiation entering from around the edges of the lenses.
   2. Watch. A watch with a second hand or one that clearly shows the seconds, or a timer is *mandatory*.
   3. Tape measure:
      a. *Never* estimate the distance. A tape measure is *mandatory* to measure the distance between the source of the ultraviolet and the highest area to be treated.
      b. A steel tape measure or one of unstretchable material is preferable.
      c. Some lamps have a tape measure built into the lamp on the outside of the hood at the level of the tube.
   4. Drape sheets or preferably a cotton bath blanket.

G. Exposure times to use for each area if the patient is treated every other day:
   1. First treatment. Use the patient's MED time.
   2. Second treatment. Double the MED time or increase by fifteen seconds.
   3. Third treatment. Triple the MED time or increase by thirty seconds.
   4. When a weekend intervenes, use the same exposure time as that used for the treatment on Friday.
   5. If one week or more passes between treatments, use the original MED time when resuming treatments.

## II. Starting the Treatment

A. *This procedure requires practice on the part of the patient.* A good time to practice is when the patient comes in for the necessary MED test. After the test has been completed, shut off the lamp and have the patient go through the procedure several times.
B. When exposing the entire body:
   1. Use four exposures on an adult — upper half of the body and then the lower half when the patient is prone (supine), and then repeat on the other side.
   2. A child may be treated with one exposure on both the front and back of the body.
C. Explain the procedure to the patient. Reassure him that the treatment booth curtains will be completely closed.
D. Instruct the patient to:
   1. Completely undress.
   2. Get onto the table on his back (stomach).
   3. Cover himself with the bath blanket (sheet).
   4. Call you when he is ready.
E. Provide the patient with goggles. Goggles are *absolutely mandatory* for the patient during this procedure.
F. Bring the lamp over the patient. Measure and center the lamp (see General Exposure).
G. Be *sure* the patient's goggles are in place.
H. With the bath blanket still completely covering the patient,

open the shutters.

I.  Leave the treatment booth, and make sure the curtains will remain completely closed. Either hold them shut, or use a snap clothespin, safety pin, etc.

J.  Tell the patient to grasp the drape blanket at his head but not to uncover himself until you tell him to do so.

K.  A few seconds before you start timing, tell the patient to uncover himself to the appropriate level. From previous practice, he should know what this level is and in which position to place his arms during the treatment.

L.  A few seconds before the time is up, tell him to grasp the blanket and get ready to cover himself completely, including his head.

M.  At the end of the time, the patient pulls up the blanket.

N.  When the patient is covered, go into the booth and close the lamp shutters.

### III. Terminating the Treatment

A.  If another patient is to follow within twenty minutes, leave the lamp on to avoid the necessary cooling and reheating time. If the lamp is turned off, open the shutters to allow faster cooling. Some lamps cannot be restarted until they have cooled.

B.  Turn off the lamp and move it to the back of the treatment booth out of the patient's way.

C.  Remove the patient's goggles.

D.  Tell the patient:
    1.  He can expect a mild sunburn.
    2.  It should appear in from six to twelve hours.

E.  That patient's record should include:
    1.  Date of the treatment.
    2.  The exposure time used.
    3.  The distance from the source to the patient.
    4.  Specific lamp used. Identify the lamp by the serial number, color, etc.

## Chapter 27

# ULTRAVIOLET AND COAL TAR

## *I. Preparations:*

A. Determine the procedure to be used:
   1. Techniques:
      a. The coal tar ointment is applied to the skin before treatment. Immediately prior to the treatment, most of the ointment is removed with olive oil. The skin should retain a brown stain appearance.
      b. Or the coal tar is washed off with soap and water.
      c. Do *not* apply coal tar to the face.
B. The patient's minimal erythemal dose (MED) time using coal tar *must* be known. The MED time should be rechecked:
   1. At least every six months.
   2. If the skin to be treated has changed color since the last treatment.
   3. If the patient is now getting sensitizers:
      a. Drugs such as sulfa, quinine, or the tetracyclene group.
      b. Endocrines such as insulin or thyroxine.
      c. Heavy metals such as gold.
   4. If the patient is getting these sensitizers, reduce the MED test times.
C. Check the lamp:
   1. Usually a general lamp is used.
   2. Know how to operate the lamp and the manual adjustments.
   3. Do *not* use the lamp if the shutters are not working properly.
   4. The quartz tube, hood and shutter reflectors should be clean and dust free:

225

      a. Do *not* touch the tube with your fingers as perspiration can damage the tube.

      b. Use Bon Ami, distilled water or absolute alcohol. Do *not* use rubbing alcohol or abrasives.

    5. Know where the tube is attached to the hood as this attachment is used as a reference point for measuring the distance between the source of the radiation and the skin.

D.  Warm up the lamp *before* the patient comes in:

    1. The shutters *must* remain tightly closed during the warm-up period and until timing actually begins.

    2. If using a combination ultraviolet/infrared lamp, turn on the correct switch.

    3. The warm-up time is usually five to ten minutes depending on the number of hours the tube has been used.

    4. *Never* cover the lamp hood as it will get hot, and the covering could catch fire. Some radiation will escape where the shutters meet.

E.  Have all materials ready to use:

    1. Goggles. Regular eyeglasses or dark glasses are *not* acceptable. They will shut out the harmful radiation that comes directly at them; however, radiation can reach the eyes by coming in around the edges of the lenses.

    2. Watch. A watch with a second hand or one that shows the seconds continuously is *mandatory* as timing must be accurate. As treatment times lengthen, a timer may be used.

    3. Tape measure. A tape measure is necessary to measure the distance between the source of the ultraviolet and the highest area to be treated:

      a. *Never* estimate the spacing.

      b. A steel tape measure or one made of unstretchable material is preferable.

      c. Some lamps have a tape measure built into them on the outside of the hood at the level of the quartz tube.

    4. Drape sheets.

## II. *Starting the Treatment*

A. Exposure times. The erythema should have subsided before treating the patient. If the patient is treated every other day:
   1. First treatment. Use the patient's first degree erythemal dose time if the area to be treated is large. A second degree erythema may be given to a small area.
   2. Second treatment. Double the time.
   3. Third treatment. Triple the time.
   4. When a weekend intervenes, use the same exposure time that was used on Friday.
   5. If one week intervenes, use the original time.
   6. Timing routines will vary depending on the skin condition.
B. Explain the procedure to the patient:
   1. Tell him that he should get a sunburn as he did after the MED test and that the area may be a little tender.
   2. Explain why he is being treated.
   3. Tell him his eyes must be protected as well as other areas not being treated, and tell him why.
   4. If you use the word *radiation,* reassure the patient that ultraviolet radiation is not the same as atomic radiation.
C. The therapist should stay out of the radiation as much as possible.
D. Check the skin.
E. Remove the coal tar:
   1. If the patient is an inpatient, this could be done by the nursing staff in the patient's room immediately before he is brought to the department.
   2. If he is an outpatient:
      a. Put on some gloves and remove the coal tar with olive oil or soap and water.
      b. If the coal tar covers a large area of the patient's body, have the patient take a shower if possible.
E. Proceed with the treatment as described in Chapter 25 General Exposure.

### III. Terminating the Treatment

A. If another patient is to follow within twenty minutes, leave the lamp on to avoid the necessary cooling and reheating times. If the lamp is accidentally turned off, open the shutters to allow faster cooling. Most lamps cannot be restarted until they have cooled. The time required for a lamp to cool depends on the ambient temperature.

B. Turn off the lamp and move it to the back of the treatment cubicle out of the patient's way.

C. Remove the patient's goggles.

D. Tell the patient:
   1. He can expect a sunburn.
   2. It should appear in two to six hours.
   3. Tell the patient to report to you any itching of the treated skin. If this occurs, reduce the exposure times or use the *same* exposure time you used for the last treatment.

E. The patient's record should include:
   1. Date of the treatment.
   2. Exposure time used.
   3. The distance from the source of the ultraviolet to the skin.
   4. Specific lamp used.

# Part VII
# Traction Techniques

*Chapter 28*

# MANUAL CERVICAL TRACTION

## *I. Preparations*

A. Determine the procedure to be used:
  1. Select the type of traction:
    a. Dynamic traction. The patient performs active neck exercises while constant traction is applied, or the traction is applied intermittently with no exercises being done.
    b. Static traction. Traction is applied continually without pauses.
  2. Check the unit:
    a. Be sure the pulleys and ropes or cables are intact.
    b. The head halter and straps should be clean and safe.
  3. Put the chair (unit) in the proper position:
    a. The patient's head should be in twenty to thirty degrees of flexion when he is in traction.
    b. The chair or unit should be placed so the free suspended rope or cable falls immediately in front of the patient's head and in the exact center of his head.
B. Have all materials ready to use:
  1. Gauze or tissue to cover the head halter for hygienic and padding purposes.
  2. A pillow for the patient's lap on which he may rest his forearms.
  3. A footstool if the chair is too high.
  4. Water in which to place dentures.

## *II. Starting the Treatment*

A. Explain the procedure to the patient:

1. Explain why the treatment is being done.
2. Explain the head halter:
    a. Show him where the pressure points will be.
    b. Tell him that the halter will be snug but not tight.
3. Tell him what he should feel and show him where he should feel it:
    a. The sensation should be a gentle pull.
    b. He should feel most of the pressure on the occiput.
    c. He should feel very little pressure on his chin, and he will not feel anything around his neck.
4. Explain the type of traction you will use and the exercises he is to perform.

B.  Ask the patient to tell you if he feels:
    1. Increased pain in the cervical area.
    2. Any radiating pain down one or both arms.
    3. Dizziness, numbness in his hand/fingers, etc.

C.  Tell the patient to sit in the chair. Be *sure* he does not move the chair:
    1. When seated, the patient's feet should rest comfortably on the floor. If the chair is too high, it is important that a footstool be provided so the patient will be as relaxed as possible.
    2. Place a pillow in his lap and have him rest his forearms and elbows on it. Be sure he is not actively holding his forearms on the pillow.

D.  Put the head halter on the patient:
    1. Glasses must be removed.
    2. Ask the patient if he wears dentures. Dentures should be removed, as they might slip and injure the gums:
        a. Explain this to the patient.
        b. Provide water in which to place the dentures.
        c. Give the patient a mouth guard or a thick gauze pad to place between his gums.
    3. Wigs may have to be removed.
    4. Keep the patient's hair as neat as possible.
    5. Remove earrings.
    6. The chin pieces, mandibular and occipital straps should be padded with gauze for comfort and hygienic

purposes.

    7. Fasten the halter in place. Be *sure* the connecting or side straps are fastened securely.

E. Connect the halter to the spreader bar.

F. Connect the spreader bar to the pulley.

G. Take up the slack in the rope or cable.

H. Recheck:

    1. The angle of pull. The angle of flexion should be twenty to thirty degrees.

    2. The rope or cable should be lined up with the exact center of the patient's head.

    3. All slack should be taken out of the rope before traction is applied.

I. Reassure the patient. Some patients will be afraid they will be hanged.

J. Determine the patient's tolerance to the traction:

    1. The pull should begin slowly with gradually increasing traction to the amount desired.

    2. The patient may be able to tolerate only a few pounds of traction (10-15) initially.

K. The release should be done slowly and gradually with no jerky movements and no sudden release of the traction.

L. Active exercises may be done while the traction is on.

M. The treatment time will vary according to the patient's tolerance. Usually, fifteen minutes is sufficient.

### III. Terminating the Treatment

A. Slowly release the traction.

B. Disconnect the halter from the spreader bar.

C. Remove the halter from the patient.

D. Check the patient for nausea, light-headedness, dizziness, headache, etc. before allowing him to leave the department. If he is an outpatient and will be driving, be sure he will be able to drive safely.

E. Dispose of padding and hygienic coverings, and clean the halter if possible.

F. Record on the patient's record:

1. Approximate poundage used.
2. Time intervals between pulls.
3. Number of pulls or total treatment time.
4. Any exercises performed.
5. Any adverse reactions to the traction

## *IV. Home Use of Traction*

A.  A simple traction apparatus can be rented or purchased.
B.  The patient should bring the apparatus to the department and learn how to use it *before* he uses it at home:
   1. Instruct him in the exact placement of the chair.
   2. Tell him how long to use the traction at any one time.
   3. Tell him how many times a day/week to use the traction.
   4. Tell him what he should not feel.
   5. Have him do the *entire* procedure by himself at least twice under your guidance.

## Chapter 29

# MOTORIZED CERVICAL TRACTION

## *I. Preparations*

A. Select the type of traction:
   1. Dynamic traction. The patient performs active neck exercises while constant traction is applied, or the traction is applied intermittently without exercises being done.
   2. Static traction. Traction is applied constantly for a period of time without pauses.
B. Select the patient's position:
   1. Sitting:
      a. This position is more convenient for the therapist as it requires less preparation than does the supine position.
      b. The patient's body weight is used as countertraction.
   2. Supine:
      a. In this position, the patient is usually more relaxed and less apprehensive.
      b. The traction can be applied for a longer period of time.
      c. There is more body stabilization.
C. Check the unit:
   1. The unit should be grounded.
   2. Know how to operate the unit.
   3. Set all dials to zero.
   4. Allow the unit to warm up if necessary.
   5. Be *sure* the head halter, straps, cable and halter fastenings are secure.
D. If the patient is sitting, put the chair (unit) in the correct position:
   1. The chair or unit should be placed so the free suspended cable falls immediately in front of the patient's

head and in the exact center.

2. The patient's head should be in twenty to thirty degrees of flexion when he is in traction.

E. Have all necessary materials ready to use:
    1. Tissue, gauze or toweling to cover the head halter for hygienic and padding purposes.
    2. Pillow to put in the patient's lap for his forearms.
    3. Water for dentures.
    4. Footstool.
    5. Mouth guard.

## II. Starting the Treatment

A. Explain the procedure to the patient:
    1. Explain why the treatment is being done.
    2. Explain the head halter:
      a. Show him where the pressure points will be.
      b. Explain that the halter will be snug but not tight.
    3. Tell him what he should feel and show him where he should feel it:
      a. The sensation should be a pull.
      b. He should feel most of the pressure on the occiput.
      c. He should feel very little pressure on his chin.
    4. Explain the type of traction the patient will get:
      a. If using continuous traction, explain this to the patient and tell him how long he will be in traction.
      b. If using intermittent traction, describe the sensation. Tell him how long the traction will be on and off during each cycle and the total treatment time.

B. Ask the patient to tell you if he feels:
    1. Increased pain in the cervical area.
    2. Any radiating pain down one or both arms.
    3. Dizziness, numbness in his hands/fingers, etc.

C. Place the patient in the predetermined position:
    1. Whether sitting or supine, twenty to thirty degrees of neck flexion is necessary while the patient is in traction.

2. If the patient is sitting:
    a. Use a chair and not a stool.
    b. Warn the patient not to move the chair as he sits down, and tell him why.
    c. The patient's feet should rest comfortably on the floor. If the chair is too high, provide a footstool.
    d. The patient should be sitting erect with his back against the backrest.
    e. One or two pillows in the patient's lap on which he may rest his forearms and elbows may allow him to relax.
3. If the patient is supine:
    a. Place one or two pillows under the knees.
    b. Be sure the patient is warm.
D. Put the head halter on the patient:
    1. Glasses must be removed.
    2. Ask the patient if he wears dentures. Dentures should be removed, as they might slip and injure the gums:
        a. Explain this to the patient.
        b. Provide water in which to place the dentures.
        c. Give the patient a mouth guard or a thick gauze pad to put between his gums.
    3. Wigs may have to be removed.
    4 Keep the patient's hair as neat as possible.
    5. Remove earrings.
    6. The chin piece, mandibular and occipital straps should be padded with gauze for comfort and hygienic purposes.
    7. Fasten the halter in place. Be *sure* the connecting or side straps are fastened securely.
E. Connect the halter to the spreader bar.
F. Connect the spreader bar to the traction unit cable.
G. Recheck:
    1. The angle of pull. The angle should *never* be zero and the head should *never* be in extension.
    2. The position of the cable to be sure it is lined up with the exact center of the patient's head.

3. To be sure all slack is out of the cable before traction is applied.
4. All halter fastenings to be sure they are secure.
H. Be *sure* the poundage dial is at zero before activating the unit.
I. Set the timer for the desired time ratio. Usually one minute on and thirty seconds off is satisfactory.
J. Set the poundage control for the desired poundage. Ten pounds may be all the patient can tolerate for the first or first few treatments.
K. Set the treatment time for twenty to thirty minutes.
L. For at least the first treatment, the therapist should remain with the patient perhaps throughout the treatment or at least until determining the traction pull is appropriate and tolerable for the patient, etc.
M. Check back frequently to be sure all is well.

## III. Terminating the Treatment

A. During the last thirty seconds of treatment, gradually reduce the tension to avoid a sudden shut-off by the automatic timer.
B. Turn all dials back to zero.
C. Remove the spreader bar and halter.
D. Evaluate the patient for nausea, dizziness, headache, etc. before allowing him to leave the department. If he is an outpatient and will be driving, be *sure* he can drive safely.
E. Return the patient's glasses, dentures, etc.
F. Dispose of padding and hygienic coverings.
G. Record on the patient's record:
    1. Poundage used.
    2. Time on/off.
    3. Total treatment time.
    4. Any exercises performed.
    5. Any adverse reaction to treatment. Reduce the poundage and/or length of the next treatment if the patient experienced any discomfort. If pain continues, discontinue treatment until the physician has been notified.

## Chapter 30

# MOTORIZED PELVIC TRACTION

## *I. Preparations*

A.  Set up the unit.
B.  Check the unit to be used:
    1.  The unit should be grounded.
    2.  Know how to operate the unit.
    3.  Set all dials to zero.
    4.  Warm up the unit if necessary.
    5.  Set the unit for intermittent or continuous traction. Intermittent is usually used.
    6.  Set the unit for the desired number of pounds. Fifty to one hundred pounds is usually sufficient.
C.  Check the pelvic belt, restraint harness, etc. for safety.
D.  Prepare the treatment setup:
    1.  If the traction unit is separate from the table, it is preferable to use a cart for the patient as it is usually higher than the average treatment table. The cart must be locked in place.
    2.  Lay the pelvic belt in the approximate position on the cart.
    3.  Countertraction may be necessary if the pelvic traction is sufficient to cause the patient to slide on the table.
    4.  If possible, the foot of the table should be raised 4 to 6 inches. If this is not possible, use pillows under the patient's knees and calves to flatten the lumbar spine as much as possible.

## *II. Starting the Treatment*

A.  Explain the procedure to the patient:
    1.  Tell him why the treatment is being done.
    2.  Explain the pelvic belt and restraint harness or strap:

       a. Tell him why these must be worn.

       b. Explain that these straps must be snug to prevent them from slipping.

    3. Tell him what he should feel and where he should feel it:

       a. The sensation should be a pull.

       b. He should feel it around the iliac crests.

B.  Ask the patient to tell you if he feels:

    1. A sudden or sharp pain.

    2. Pain radiating down his leg(s).

    3. Any numbness in his leg(s).

C.  Explain the type of traction he will get:

    1. If using intermittent traction, describe the sensation. Tell him how long the traction will be on and off during each cycle.

    2. If using continuous traction, tell him how long he will be in traction.

    3. Tell him the total treatment time.

D.  Have the patient lie supine on the belt and harness straps:

    1. Be sure the belt and straps are in the proper position.

    2. Be sure his hips and knees are flexed.

    3. The pelvic belt should be placed around the waist so the pull will come on the iliac crests.

    4. The restraint strap is placed above the pelvic belt below the rib cage, or use the shoulder harness.

    5. You may have to pad the belt (straps).

E.  Connect the pelvic belt to the unit.

F.  Check all fastenings and the fit of the belt for snugness.

G.  Check the angle of pull:

    1. A posterior pelvic tilt is usually used.

    2. There should be no lateral deviation.

H.  Take up all slack in both belt and harness.

I.  *Check the poundage.*

J.  Turn on the timer. Treatment time will vary from ten to thirty minutes.

K.  Activate the unit.

L.  Stay with the patient until you are sure he is tolerating the treatment with no problems.

M. Check frequently to be sure all is well.

### III. Terminating the Treatment

A. Some units will be shut off by the timer. If the unit shuts off while the traction is on, reactivate the timer and shut off the main switch after the traction is released.
B. *Turn the poundage back to zero.* Some units can be used for cervical traction. *Severe* consequences can result from using too much force on the cervical area.
C. Remove the pelvic belt and restraint straps.
D. Evaluate the patient for any untoward symptoms.
E. Record on the patient's record:
    1. The poundage used.
    2. Time on/off.
    3. Total treatment time.
    4. Any adverse reaction. If the patient experienced any discomfort, reduce the poundage and/or length of the next treatment. If these measures do not provide any relief, discontinue treatment.

# Part VIII
# Miscellaneous Techniques

## Chapter 31

# CONTRAST BATHS

## I. *Preparations*

A. Select the timing routine. Timing routines may vary, but they should be exact:
   1. Always start with *hot* and end with *hot*.
   2. Examples of timing routines:
      a. Three minutes in hot and one minute in cold; alternate for thirty-one minutes.
      b. Four minutes in hot and one minute in cold; alternate for twenty-eight minutes.
      c. Five minutes in hot and two minutes in cold; alternate for thirty-three minutes.
B. Set up the treatment where hot and cold water or ice are readily available to maintain the bath temperatures throughout the treatment time.
C. You will need two containers large enough to immerse the parts to be treated. Large plastic or polyethylene wastebaskets may be used for the lower extremities.
D. Fill the clean containers two-thirds full of water:
   1. Do *not* fill the containers too full as immersion of the extremities will cause the water to overflow.
   2. The water temperature in one container should be between 55° and 65° F.
   3. The water temperature in the other container should be between 95° and 105° F.
   4. Add a disinfectant to the water if the patient has an open or infected lesion.
E. Several turkish towels and possibly a drape sheet will be needed.

## II. *Starting the Treatment*

A. Advanced arteriosclerosis and advanced peripheral vascular disease should be treated with *extreme* caution if at all.

B. If the lower extremities are to be treated:
1. Provide a chair low (high) enough to allow the patient's feet to rest comfortably on the bottoms of the containers when immersed.
2. Or elevate the containers.
3. The containers should not be too tall as the edges may cause pressure points under the knees.

C. Explain the procedure to the patient:
1. One container contains hot water and the other contains cold water. Tell him what the water temperatures are and that the hot water is not hot enough to burn him. Demonstrate by putting your hand into the hot water, or allow him to feel of the water if necessary.
2. A time routine must be followed. Explain what you want him to do and the timing routine to be followed.
3. Immersion into one container from the other must be immediate and complete, and tell him why.
4. He should let you know if any discomfort occurs.

D. Instruct the patient to remove the appropriate clothing. Provide him with necessary draping, etc.

E. Remove his watch if appropriate.

F. Protect his remaining clothing and the floor from the water.

G. Inspect the skin to be treated.

H. Instruct (help) the patient to immerse the part(s) into the hot water.

I. At the end of the desired time, instruct the patient to remove the part from the hot water and immediately immerse it into the cold water:
1. You should remain with the patient until you are confident he will follow the timing routine exactly.
2. Provide him with a watch or timer.

J. Maintain the correct water temperatures:
1. If hot water needs to be added during the treatment, *always* remove the extremity before adding the water.

2. Recheck the water temperatures with a thermometer and your hand if ice or hot water is added.
K. Keep the patient warm throughout the treatment.

### III. Terminating the Treatment

A. Remove the extremity and have (help) the patient dry himself.
B. Check the skin.
C. Wipe up any water on the floor before allowing the patient to move from the area.

### IV. Notes

A. Home use of contrast baths:
   1. Tell the patient about using plastic wastebaskets.
   2. Write down:
      a. The water temperatures for each container.
      b. The timing routine he is to follow.
      c. How many times a day he should use the baths.
      d. How many times a week he should use the baths.
   3. Instruct him to always check the water temperature with his hand and a candy or dairy thermometer.
B. Containers should be washed with a mild disinfectant and soap after each treatment.

## Chapter 32

# TANK OR POOL HOIST

## I. Starting the Treatment

A. Determine the procedure to be used.
B. Check the hoist:
  1. Know how to operate the unit.
  2. The hoist should be grounded.
  3. Test it to be sure it is operating safely and efficiently.
  4. The cables should not be frayed or twisted.
  5. Cable hooks should be working properly.
  6. Be sure the stretcher rings to which the cables will be attached are safe.
  7. The stretcher canvas must be securely attached to the frame.
C. Align the plinth with the hoist so the middle of the plinth (from end to end) is directly under the hoist track.
D. Place a safety strap on the plinth:
  1. If the patient has *any* upper extremity *and/or* neck weakness *and/or* he cannot swim, he should be secured to the stretcher with a wide strap.
  2. The strap should be between the plinth and stretcher at the approximate level of the patient's hips.
E. Place the hoist stretcher on the plinth:
  1. Be sure the holes in the stretcher frame are down.
  2. If the stretcher is wet, place two turkish towels on it in a lengthwise fashion.
F. Check the tank/pool headrest to be sure it is secure.

## II. Starting the Treatment

A. You may need assistance:
  1. When in doubt, always have another staff member ready to assist you.

2. Assistance may be required if any non weight bearing patient is going into the pool.
B. Explain the procedure to the patient:
   1. A careful and full explanation is essential.
   2. He will be placed onto the stretcher, lifted into the water, etc.
   3. Tell him the water temperature.
   4. Reassure him:
      a. The hoist is safe and he will not be dropped.
      b. Explain the safety strap and life preserver.
      c. Explain the head rest if it is to be used.
      d. Explain any exercises, turbine action, etc.
      e. Assure him that you will remain with him.
C. If the hoist is over the stretcher, move it out of the way.
D. Transfer the patient from the cart to the stretcher:
   1. The patient's position on the stretcher is *very* important. Place him more toward the *foot* end of the stretcher. If he is placed in the center or more toward the head end, the head end of the stretcher will go down as soon as the hoist lifts the patient off the plinth.
   2. Check to be sure the patient's arms, elbows and hands are completely on the stretcher.
   3. Pad any pressure points (heels and elbows) with towels if they are tender and/or are resting on the stretcher frame.
   4. A tank pillow may be used for the head.
   5. A life preserver may be indicated.
   6. Fasten the security strap:
      a. Be sure it fits securely over the pelvis and not around the waist.
      b. Some straps may shrink when they get wet.
E. Slide the hoist over the patient. Do not allow the cables to touch the patient.
F. Connect the cables to the stretcher:
   1. Hold all four cables in one hand.
   2. Lower the crossbar sufficiently to allow the cables to reach each corner of the stretcher.

3. The shortest cables (if available) should be toward the patient's head. If the cables are even in length, the patient must be placed more toward the foot end of the stretcher.
4. Be sure the cables are not crossed or twisted.
5. The open ends of the cable hooks should be directed outward.
6. Connect the cables. *Never take the head end cables over the patient's face.*

G. Raise the crossbar only enough to take the slack out of the cables.
H. Recheck to be *sure* the snap hooks are securely locked on the ends of the stretcher rings.
I. Warn the patient that he is about to be lifted.
J. Raise the stretcher to a height sufficient to allow the patient's hips to clear the tank or pool edge:
1. Guide the stretcher with one hand:
a. Do *not* let it swing.
b. If the stretcher has a tendency to swing, it was not placed correctly in relation to the hoist track originally.
2. When raised, the stretcher should be level, or preferably the foot end should be down slightly. If the head end is down, lower the stretcher onto the plinth and move the patient further down toward the foot end.

K. If necessary, turn the stretcher to align it with the hoist track:
1. Turn the stretcher slowly.
2. Any jerks or fast movement will increase the patient's apprehension.
L. Move the hoist smoothly and slowly along the track to the desired position. Use good body mechanics.
M. Warn the patient that he is about to be lowered into the water:
1. Stand by his head.
2. Remind him that the water is warm.
3. Assure him he will not float off the stretcher.
4. Assure him that the head (stretcher) rest is secure.

N. Lower the patient into the water:
 1. As the stretcher is lowered, guide it onto the head rest and make *absolutely certain* that it is secure.
 2. Remove any towels used for padding.
O. Lower the crossbar to allow removal of the cables:
 1. The cables may be left attached to the stretcher to provide more security for the patient.
 2. If the patient is to be removed from the stretcher, the cables should be removed first.
P. Remove the cables.
O. Hold onto the cables, raise the crossbar and move the hoist out of the way.

### III. Terminating the Treatment

A. Place towels or a bath blanket on the plinth.
B. Be sure the patient is more toward the foot end of the stretcher.
C. Return the hoist to the center position over the stretcher.
D. Hold onto the cables, and lower the crossbar sufficiently to allow the cables to reach each corner of the stretcher:
 1. The cables should not touch the patient.
 2. The shortest cables should be toward the patient's head.
 3. The cables should not be crossed or twisted.
 4. The open ends of the cable hooks should be directed out.
 5. Attach the cables. Do *not* take the cables over the patient's face.
E. Raise the crossbar only enough to take any slack out of the cables.
F. Recheck to be sure all cables are secure.
G. Warn the patient that he is about to be lifted out of the water.
H. Guiding the stretcher with one hand, raise the patient out of the water. Be sure the stretcher is high enough above the water to allow the patient's hips to clear the edge of the tank or pool.
I. As soon as the stretcher clears the water:

1. Warn the patient.
2. Tilt the stretcher slightly (foot end down) to allow the excess water to drain from the holes in the stretcher frame.
3. After most of the excess water has drained:
   a. Cover the patient with a bath blanket or towels.
   b. If the room temperature is below 85° F, cover the patient as soon as he is raised out of the water.

J. Guiding the stretcher with one hand, slide the stretcher along the track to a position over the plinth.
   1. Avoid jerky movements.
   2. Use good body mechanics.

K. If necessary, turn the stretcher *slowly* to align it with the plinth.

L. Warn the patient that he is about to be lowered onto the plinth:
   1. Check to be *sure* the patient's elbows and hands are on the stretcher.
   2. The patient should *not* be holding onto the edge of the stretcher.
   3. Be sure the stretcher is level or that the foot end is down slightly.

M. Guide the stretcher and lower it onto the plinth.

N. Lower the crossbar sufficiently to loosen the cables:
   1. Watch the patient's head to be sure the cables do not touch his face.
   2. Remove the head end cables first:
      a. Do not take the cables over the patient's face.
      b. Hold onto these cables or attach them to the foot end cables.
   3. Remove the foot end cables.

O. Move the hoist away from the patient.

P. Give the patient a towel and instruct (help) him to dry himself thoroughly.

Q. *Keep the patient warm.*

*Chapter 33*

# HUBBARD TANK

## *I. Preparations*

A. The room temperature should be at least 80° F and preferably warmer.

B. Fill the clean tank with water at a temperature of 96° to
100° F.

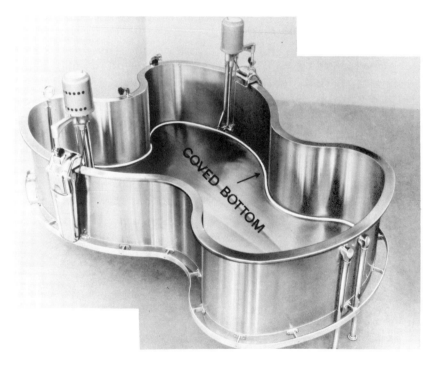

Figure 40. Hubbard tank. (Courtesy of Ille Division of Market Forge)

C. Have all necessary materials ready to use:

    1. Bathing suit, T-binder, or other appropriate clothing.

2. Turkish towels.
3. Cotton bath blanket.
4. Splints, braces, weights, etc.
5. Cephalic cold and tepid drinking water should be readily available.
D. Check the equipment to be used:
1. Be sure the hoist is operating safely and efficiently.
2. Test the turbines if they are going to be used.
3. Be sure the tank headrest is secure.

## II. Starting the Treatment

A. The patient must be medically cleared before treatment:
1. Colds, sore throats, rashes, infections, etc. are contraindications for treatment.
2. *Never* put a cardiac or respiratory patient into the tank.
B. The patient should evacuate bowels and bladder before being put into the tank:
1. If the patient has an indwelling catheter, be sure you know the nursing or doctor's procedure for handling the catheter *before* you place the patient in the water.
C. Explain the procedure to the patient:
1. He should know why he is being treated in the water.
2. Tell him the water temperature is warm.
3. Explain the hoist.
4. Explain the action of the turbines if they are to be used.
5. Tell him the depth of the water.
6. Show him the headrest and its stability.
7. Reassure him:
   a. You should remain at the patient's side at least for the first few treatments, depending on the treatment procedure.
   b. *Never* leave the immediate vicinity even for a few *seconds.*
D. Instruct (help) the patient to completely undress and to put on a bathing suit, T-binder or other appropriate clothing. Be sure the patient is properly draped at all times.
E. Remove all jewelry, dressings, etc.

F.  The patient should provide his own bathing cap if he wants one.
G.  *If the patient has any upper extremity and/or neck weakness and/or he cannot swim, have him wear a life jacket* (not a life belt) or strap him to the hoist stretcher.
H.  If the patient is non weight bearing, use the hoist to put him into the water.
I.  Be *sure* the patient's head is secure.
J.  Allow the patient to adjust to the water *before* exercising or turning on the turbine(s). This may take several treatments.
K.  One "slip" in handling the patient will make him extremely apprehensive.
L.  Perform exercises:
    1.  The turbine may be on or off.
    2.  Good body mechanics are essential for you. It may be easier and safer for you to go into the tank with the patient to perform exercises depending on the type of tank you are using.
M.  Treatment time is usually twenty to thirty minutes.
N.  If the patient becomes overheated, tired, dizzy or if any untoward symptoms develop, terminate treatment.
O.  If a bowel movement occurs, as can happen with spinal cord injury patients, remove the patient from the water immediately and clean the tank.

### III. Terminating the Treatment

A.  Remove the patient from the water and allow (help) him to dry himself thoroughly.
B.  Allow him to dress or cover him with a bath blanket, and move him to a plinth for further treatment. *Keep the patient warm.*
C.  If you have been treating an outpatient, suggest he remain in the waiting room for twenty minutes to cool off before going outside.
D.  Drain and clean the tank. Check to be sure there are no dressings, tape, etc. in the water before draining the tank.

*IV. Notes*

To sterilize the tank:
A.  Completely drain the tank.
B.  Put the hoist stretcher, headrest, cable hooks, splints, etc. in the bottom of the tank.
C.  Scrub all equipment with a brush dipped in Zephiran® Chloride.
D.  Fill the tank with water at 115° F or hotter to above the turbine intakes (if the turbine was used or was in the water).
E.  Add 8 ounces of Zephiran Chloride.
F.  Run the turbine for four minutes.
G.  While the turbine is running, wash the insides of the tank, turbine tubes, etc.
H.  Turn off the turbine and wash its undersides and up into the tubes.
I.  Leave the equipment in the tank and drain the tank.
J.  Fill the tank with the hottest water possible to cover the equipment in the tank.
K.  Let the water stand for ten minutes.
L.  Add cold water to cool down the temperature.
M.  Rinse down the equipment and insides of the tank.
N.  Drain the tank and remove all equipment.
O.  Soak a sponge in Zephiran Chloride and wash the agitator and sides of the tank.
P.  Allow the tank to dry.

## Chapter 34

# THERAPEUTIC POOL

## *I. Preparations*

A.  The temperature of the pool *room* should be at least 80° F and preferably warmer.
B.  Check the water temperature. Ninety-six to ninety-eight degrees Fahrenheit is recommended.
C.  Have all necessary equipment ready:
    1. Bathing suits, T-binders or other appropriate clothing.
    2. Turkish towels.
    3. Large cotton bath blankets.
    4. Life belts.
    5. Life jackets.
    6. Hoist.
    7. Plinth.
    8. Splints, floats, weights, etc.
D.  The water chlorine content should be checked according to public health requirements. Twice daily is recommended.
E.  Bacterial testing should be done weekly.
F.  Emptying and cleaning of the pool should be done regularly depending on the pool size and usage.

## *II. Starting the Treatment*

A.  The patient must be medically cleared before treatment:
    1. Colds, sore throats, rashes and infections are contraindications for treatment.
    2. *Never* put a cardiac or respiratory patient into the pool.
    3. Incontinent patients should be treated in a tank.
B.  The patient should evacuate bowels and bladder before treatment.
C.  The patient should be clean.
D.  Instruct (help) the patient to completely undress and to put

257

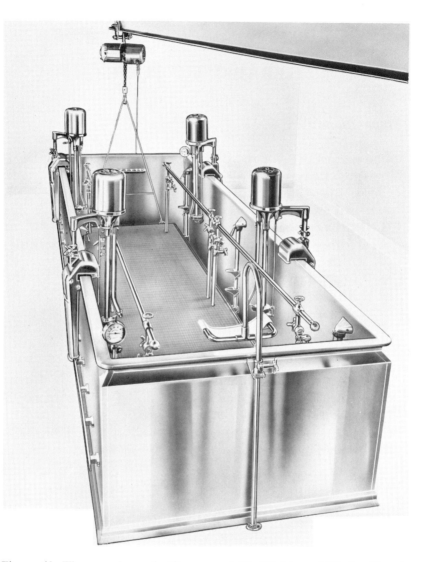

Figure 41. Therapeutic pool. (Courtesy of Ille Division of Market Forge)

  on a bathing suit, T-binder, or other appropriate clothing. Be sure the patient is properly draped at all times.

E. Remove all jewelry, dressings, tape, etc.

F. The patient should provide a bathing cap if he wants one.

G. Cotton or paper scuffers should be available for the patient to get from the dressing room to the pool.

H. Explain the procedure to the patient:
   1. You will be in the pool with him at all times.
   2. Explain why he is being treated in the pool.
   3. Show him any equipment you will use.
   4. Explain the hoist.
   5. Tell him the water is warm.
   6. Reassure him.

I. *If the patient has any upper extremity and/or neck weakness and/or he cannot swim, have him wear a life jacket.* A life belt will *not* keep the patient's head out of the water if he slips, etc.

J. Any braces and splints should be applied *before* the patient enters the pool.

K. If the patient is non weight bearing, use the hoist to put him into the water.

L. *The therapist must go into the pool with the patient:*
   1. The therapist should be *in* the pool before the patient goes in, and he should not leave the water until the patient is out.
   2. If the therapist cannot swim well, he should *never* treat any patient in the pool by himself, and he should *always* wear a life jacket (*not* a life belt).
   3. The therapist should never treat more than one completely disabled patient at one time.
   4. Group treatment is possible only after partially disabled patients have gained confidence in the therapist; three or four partially disabled patients are sufficient for one therapist depending on the extent of their disabilities and the therapist's ability to swim. *Never take chances with the patient's life or your own.*
   5. Each therapist should spend no more than one to one and a half hours per each half day in a pool as the warm water is very debilitating.
   6. *Never* go into the pool if you are tired or if you have any of the contraindications listed for the patient.

M. Allow the patient to adjust to the water:

1. It may take several treatments for the patient to adjust to the water.
2. It may take quite a while for the patient to gain confidence in you to the point where he will be completely relaxed and able to do what you ask him to do.
3. One "slip" in handling the patient who cannot swim and/or one who has even minor neck and/or upper extremity weakness will make the patient extremely apprehensive. The use of a life jacket with these patients cannot be overemphasized.

N. Perform exercises, gait training, etc.
O. Treatment time may be from five to thirty minutes. If the patient becomes too tired, dizzy, hot, etc., terminate treatment.

### III. Terminating the Treatment

A. Remove the patient from the water.
B. Remove exercise splints, weights, etc.
C. Do *not* allow the patient to become chilled:
   1. Stretcher patients should be covered with a bath blanket as soon as they are lifted out of the water.
   2. Bathrobes should be provided for other patients.
D. Instruct (help) the patient to dry himself thoroughly.
E. Instruct (help) the patient to dress.
F. If he is an outpatient, urge him to remain in the waiting room for twenty minutes to cool off before going outside if the outside temperature is colder than the pool room temperature.
G. Wipe up any water from the floor.

*Chapter 35*

# PHONOPHORESIS

## *I. Preparations*

A. Determine the procedure to be used:
   1. The contact technique must be used (see Chap. 8).
   2. Use continuous ultrasound.
   3. A moving or stationary transducer may be used:
      a. If the transducer is 13 cm² or less, the transducer should be kept in constant motion on the skin from the time the intensity is increased until the unit shuts off.
      b. A stationary transducer may be used with a 50 cm² or larger transducer.
B. Check the unit:
   1. The unit must be grounded.
   2. Know how to operate the unit.
   3. All switches and controls should be off.
   4. The transducer and plug connections should be secure.
   5. The face of the transducer should be clean.
   6. Do *not* use a unit that is not operating properly.
   7. The transducer cable should be intact.
   8. Make *sure* the intensity control is off, and warm up the unit if necessary.
C. Have all materials ready to use:
   1. Coupling medium. The substance to be introduced into the tissues is usually incorporated into the coupling medium.
   2. Turkish towels, drape sheet, etc.

## *II. Starting the Treatment*

A. If the patient complains of pain during the treatment:
   1. The first thing to do is to turn the intensity back to

zero, add more coupling medium and resume treatment.

2. If pain persists, reduce the intensity.

3. If these steps fail to stop the pain, terminate treatment.

B. *Never* treat *any* part of *any* patient who has an external or implanted atomic or electrical stimulating device of any kind. The high frequency current in the transducer cable may alter the operation of the device.

C. If you are sensitive to the drug being introduced, wear rubber gloves.

D. Explain the procedure to the patient:

   1. Tell him how long the treatment will be.

   2. Tell him he may not feel anything.

   3. Emphasize that he should tell you *immediately* if he has *any* pain in the area being treated.

   4. Show the patient the coupling medium and explain its use.

E. Check the area to be treated:

   1. The skin should be clean, dry and free from lotions, creams, etc.

   2. Check skin sensation. If sensation is lacking or diminished, use low intensity.

   3. Avoid treating on abrasions, new skin, recent scar tissue, etc.

   4. Do *not* treat on bony prominences.

   5. Do *not* treat over or near the heart.

   6. If treating a large area, divide it into sections and treat each section separately:

      a. When using a 13 cm² or smaller transducer, the treatment area should be no more than 6 by 6 inches. The smaller the transducer, the smaller the area can be.

      b. When using a 50 cm² *moving* transducer, the treatment area may be 12 by 12 inches.

      c. When using a 50 cm² *stationary* transducer, the treatment area must be the same size as the transducer.

F. Tell the patient you are going to put the cream (lotion, gel) onto his skin and that it will feel cold.

G. Apply *room temperature* or cooler coupling medium *liberally* and directly onto the skin:
1. Protect any remaining clothing from the coupling medium.
2. Be sure the patient is not sensitive to the coupling medium. This may not be discovered until after the first treatment.
3. *Never* warm up the coupling medium. When the coupling medium and transducer are cool, more heat is lost through the skin, and the deep temperature will be higher.
4. Too much coupling medium is better than too little.
5. Warm the patient and using the transducer, spread the coupling medium over the skin. Do not allow the medium to touch any of the skin not being treated.
6. It is essential that the face of the transducer be completely covered with the coupling medium.
7. Do *not* place the coupling medium container on top of the unit.

H. Recheck to be sure the intensity control is off.
I. Turn on the unit (unless preheated).
J. Set the automatic timer to the desired treatment time. The treatment time will vary depending on the intensity used. Five minutes is usually sufficient.
K. To increase the intensity with moving transducer:
1. Recheck to be sure there is enough coupling medium on the skin and transducer.
2. Apply the transducer to the skin:
   a. Transducer pressure should be firm but *not* heavy. Unless using a small transducer, usually the weight of the transducer will cause enough pressure.
   b. Complete contact is essential.
   c. The transducer *must* be held at a *right angle* to the skin being treated and the right angle must be maintained *throughout* the treatment.
3. With the transducer *constantly moving* in any direction and in firm contact with the skin, quickly adjust the

intensity control to the desired watts per centimeter squared (or total watts as indicated by the manufacturer of the unit you are using):

    a. The 13 cm² or smaller transducer *cannot* remain stationary while adjusting the intensity. (With some units, the intensity may be set while the transducer is in its holder.)

    b. If the treatment is for five minutes, the intensity is usually 1 w/cm² or less.

    c. Be *sure* to read the correct meter scale. The lower scale is usually w/cm².

L. Treatment using a moving transducer:

    1. If you have used your dominant hand to increase the intensity, quickly transfer the transducer to that hand.

    2. Constantly move the transducer in either small circles or short, longitudinal strokes:

        a. The speed of the movement is *slow* — about 1 inch per second.

        b. The next stroke should cover 50 percent of the previous stroke. Do *not* stroke forward and back in the same place or make a second circle in the same place as the previous circle.

M. To increase the intensity when the transducer is stationary:

    1. With continuous ultrasound, a 50 cm² transducer must be used.

    2. Apply the coupling medium as with the moving transducer. A gel or a cream must be used.

    3. Position the transducer on the skin. Excellent contact and a right angle should be maintained throughout the treatment.

    4. Increase the intensity to the desired level. Read the correct meter scale.

N. *Never* hold the transducer in the air with the intensity up from zero for more than a few seconds at any one time:

    1. The face of the transducer can become hot and the patient can be burned when the transducer is placed on the skin.

    2. The transducer crystal can be damaged.

3. The glue holding the crystal to the posterior surface of the transducer face can become soft.
4. Some large transducers (50 cm²) will not become hot or damaged if the total wattage intensity is low. However, the transducer should *always* be checked for heat before continuing treatment.

O. The coupling medium *must* be kept on the skin and transducer throughout the treatment. Transducer movement will spread the coupling medium thereby enlarging the treatment area. Occasionally, tip the transducer on its edge and push the coupling medium back onto the area being treated. Do *not* hold the transducer in this position for more than a few seconds.

### III. Terminating the Treatment

A. The unit will shut off automatically at the end of the treatment time.
B. Turn the intensity control back to zero. If treatment must be discontinued before the unit shuts off, keep the transducer moving until the intensity is at zero.
C. Wipe off the coupling medium from the transducer, and replace it in its holder.
D. Move the unit to the back of the treatment cubicle out of the patient's way.
E. Wipe off the coupling medium from the patient's skin.
F. Check the patient's skin.

## Chapter 36

# COMBINED ULTRASOUND AND ELECTRICAL STIMULATION

## *I. Preparations*

A. Select continuous or pulsed ultrasound. Continuous is usually used with electrical stimulation.
B. Select the ultrasound technique:
    1. Contact technique:
        a. This technique is used on relatively smooth muscular surfaces and where some light but complete transducer pressure can be tolerated.
        b. The transducer remains in contact with the skin throughout the treatment.
        c. A coupling medium must be used between the transducer and the skin. Gel is preferred. Mineral oil is not acceptable, as it is an insulator against the current.
    2. Underwater technique:
        a. This technique is used when the surface is uneven such as the hand, elbow, knee, ankle, etc., where good transducer contact is not possible or where the area to be treated is sensitive to pressure.
        b. The part to be treated and the transducer are immersed in the water.
        c. The coupling medium is the water.
        d. The transducer is held from 1/2 to 1 inch from the skin throughout the treatment.
C. Select the current modulation and modulation rate.
D. Check the unit(s) to be used:
    1. The unit must be grounded.
    2. Know how to opeate the unit.
    3. All switches should be off. Be especially certain the

intensity controls are at zero.
4. Transducer and plug connections should be tight.
5. Do not use frayed electrode wires or loose-fitting wire tips.
6. Use wire tips that fit both the electrodes and the unit. Substitutions or makeshift connections can cause burns.
7. Soak the dispersive electrode in warm water. The transducer is the active electrode.
8. Try the current and ultrasound on yourself to be sure the unit is operating safely and efficiently.
E. Have all other materials ready to use:
1. Wood plinth. Do not use a metal plinth.
2. Turkish towels.
3. Coupling medium if the contact technique is used.

## II. Starting the Treatment

A. Explain the procedure to the patient:
1. Describe the sensation he should feel.
2. Tell him how long the treatment will be.
3. Demonstrate on yourself. Get an actual contraction.
4. It may be necessary to let the patient feel the current on an area other than that you will treat before you actually begin.
5. Emphasize that he should tell you *immediately* if he has *any* pain or burning sensation in the area being treated.
B. Check the area to be treated:
1. The skin should be clean and free from lotions, oils, creams, etc.
2. Check skin sensation. If sensation is diminished or lacking, use low intensities.
3. If treating a large area, divide it into sections and treat each section separately:
   a. When using a 13 cm$^2$ or smaller transducer, the treatment area should be no more than 6 by 6 inches.
   b. When using a 50 cm$^2$ *moving* transducer, the treat-

ment area may be 12 by 12 inches.

    c. When using a 50 cm² *stationary* transducer, the treatment area must be the same size as the transducer.

C. *Never* treat *any* part of *any* patient who has an external or implanted electrical or atomic stimulating device such as a heart pacemaker or a transcutaneous stimulator.

D. Do *not* treat:

    1. Directly over, through or near the heart.

    2. Directly over, near or through a recent or nonunion fracture site.

    3. Over, near, or through a pregnant uterus.

    4. On bony prominences.

    5. On abrasions, recent scar tissue, new skin, etc.

E. Metal and electricity:

    1. *Never* treat the patient on a metal plinth or while he is sitting in a metal chair.

    2. Remove all metal in the area to be treated. Any unremovable metal, such as a wedding ring, may be covered (contact technique) or avoided (underwater technique).

    3. Do not allow the patient to touch any metal.

F. Contact technique:

    1. Active electrode: The transducer is the active electrode.

    2. Dispersive electrode:

        a. Remove the electrode from the water. It should be at least 4 by 4 inches in size.

        b. Cover the electrode with several layers of wet gauze or cotton for hygienic purposes.

        c. Squeeze the electrode and gauze gently to remove excess water. The electrode should be wet and not damp. Too much water is better than too little. The electrode *must* be kept wet throughout the treatment.

        d. Attach a lead wire to the electrode and to the unit.

        e. Warn the patient.

        f. Place the electrode in *firm* and *complete* contact on the *same* side (left versus right) of the body as that you will be treating:

1. Use the patient's weight, light sand bags or straps to hold the electrode in place.
2. If treating the back, place the electrode under a thigh.

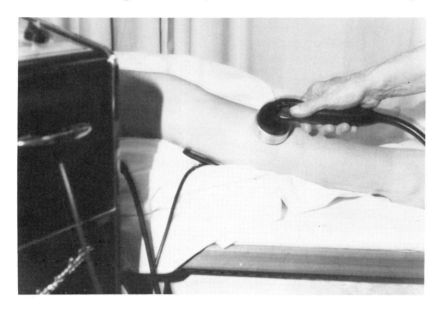

Figure 42. Combined ultrasound and electrical stimulation. (Medcosonlator by Medco Products Co.)

3. Warn the patient that you are going to put some gel (lotion) on his skin.
4. Apply *room temperature* or cooler coupling medium *liberally* and directly onto the skin:
   a. *Never* warm up the coupling medium.
   b. Too much coupling medium is better than too little.
   c. Be sure the patient is not sensitive to the coupling medium. This may not be known until after the first treatment.
   d. Protect any remaining clothing.
   e. Warn the patient, and using the transducer, spread the coupling medium over the skin.
5. Recheck to be sure the intensity control is off.

6. Turn on the unit (unless preheated).
7. Set the automatic timer to the desired treatment time. Treatment time is usually five minutes.
8. Current:
    a. With the transducer in light but complete contact, turn up the current intensity *slowly* until the patient begins to feel it.
9. Ultrasound:
    a. (see Contact Technique, Chap. 8). With the transducer in light but complete contact, *constantly moving and at a right angle to the skin,* increase the ultrasound output to 1 w/cm² or less.
10. If you have used your dominant hand to adjust the intensity, quickly transfer the transducer to that hand.
11. Constantly move the transducer in either small circles or small longitudinal strokes:
    a. The speed is *slow* — about 1 inch per second.
    b. The next circle (stroke) should cover 50 percent of the previous stroke. Do *not* stroke forward and then back in the same place or make a second circle in the same place as the first one.
12. *Never* hold the transducer in the air with the intensity up from zero for more than a few seconds at one time:
    a. The face of the transducer can become hot, and the patient can be burned when the transducer is placed on the skin.
    b. The transducer crystal can be damaged.
    c. The glue holding the crystal to the posterior surface of the transducer can become soft.
13. The coupling medium *must* be kept on the skin and the transducer throughout the treatment. Transducer movement will spread the coupling medium, thereby seemingly enlarging the treatment area. Occasionally, tip the transducer on its edge and push the coupling medium back onto the area being treated. Do *not* hold the transducer in this position for more than a few seconds at a time.
G. Underwater technique:

1. This may be done in a whirlpool with the turbine off.
2. The water temperature should be no more than 70° F.
3. The therapist should wear a rubber glove on the hand holding the transducer.
4. When air bubbles appear on the skin and/or transducer, they should be wiped away *immediately* with your hand. Putting alcohol on the skin and face of the transducer before placing them in the water will help reduce the accumulation of air bubbles.
5. Dispersive electrode:
   a. Prepare a 4 by 4 inch or larger electrode in the same manner as for the contact technique.
   b. Place the electrode on a part of the patient *outside* of the water and in *firm* and *complete* contact.
6. Have (help) the patient immerse the part in the water:
   a. The water must completely surround the part to be treated.
   b. Tell the patient not to move as this can create air bubbles in the water.
7. Slowly immerse the transducer in the water:
   a. The face of the transducer must be completely covered with water throughout the treatment.
   b. *Never* touch the skin with the transducer while the intensity is up from zero. The distance between the skin and the transducer should be from 1/2 to 1 inch.
   c. Be sure there are no air bubbles on the face of the transducer or skin before starting treatment.
8. Use the same intensities, the same transducer technique, and the same treatment time as for the contact technique.

### III. *Terminating the Treatment*

A. A few seconds *before* the automatic timer shuts the unit off, and with the transducer constantly moving, *slowly* reduce the *current* intensity to zero, and then the ultrasound intensity to zero.

B. Wipe off the coupling medium (water) from the transducer and place it in its holder.
C. Wipe off the patient's skin.
D. Remove the dispersive electrode and dry the skin.
E. Thoroughly check the patient's skin on both the treated area and under the dispersive electrode.

## Chapter 37

# TRIGGER POINT TECHNIQUE

## *I. Preparations*

A.  Select continuous or pulsed ultrasound.
B.  Use the contact technique (see Ultrasound, Contact Technique).
C.  Select the current and modulation rate.
D.  Check the unit(s) to be used:
    1. Know how to operate the unit.
    2. The unit must be grounded.
    3. All switches should be off. Be especially certain the intensity controls are off.
    4. Transducer and plug connections should be tight.
    5. Do not use frayed wires or loose-fitting wire tips.
    6. Use wire tips that fit both the electrode and the unit. Substitutions or makeshift connections can cause burns.
    7. Soak the dispersive electrode in warm water.
    8. Try the current and ultrasound on yourself to be sure the unit is operating efficiently.
E.  Have all other materials ready to use:
    1. Wood plinth. Do not use a metal plinth.
    2. Turkish towels.
    3. Coupling medium. *Do not* use mineral oil as it is an insulator against electrical currents.

## *II. Starting the Treatment*

A.  Explain the procedure to the patient:
    1. He will feel a mild prickly sensation when the current intensity is increased.
    2. If the current intensity is sufficient and a motor point is stimulated, a muscle contraction will result.

3. Instruct him to tell you when he feels a sharp, painful sensation other than the prickly sensation or the muscle contraction. This will be the trigger point. If the trigger point is stimulated, he may also feel pain in an area other than the trigger area.
4. Tell him how long the treatment will be.
5. Demonstrate on yourself. Get an actual contraction.
6. It may be necessary for you to let him feel the current on his forearm (etc.) before you treat him.

B. Check the area to be treated:
1. The skin should be clean and free from oils, creams, and lotions.
2. Check skin sensation. If sensation is lacking or diminished, use low intensities.
3. Avoid treating over abrasions, recent scar tissue or new skin.
4. Do *not* treat on bony prominences.
5. If treating a large area, divide it into sections and treat each section separately.

C. *Never* treat *any* part of *any* patient who has an external or implanted electrical or atomic stimulating device such as a heart pacemaker.

D. Do *not* treat:
1. Directly over, through or near the heart.
2. Directly over, near or through a recent or nonunion fracture site.
3. Over, near or through a pregnant uterus.

E. Metal and electricity:
1. *Never* treat the patient on a metal plinth.
2. Remove all metal in the area to be treated. Any unremovable metal should be covered with dry gauze.
3. Do *not* allow the patient to touch any metal.

F. The transducer is the active electrode.

G. The dispersive electrode:
1. Remove the electrode from the water. It should be 4 by 4 inches in size.
2. Cover the electrode with several layers of gauze or cotton for hygienic purposes.

3. Squeeze the electrode and gauze gently to remove excess water. The electrode should be wet and not damp. Too much water is better than too little. The electrode must be kept wet throughout the treatment.
4. Attach a lead wire to the electrode and to the unit.
5. Warn the patient.
6. Place the electrode in light by *complete* contact on the *same* side (left versus right) as you will be treating:
   a. Use the patient's weight, light sandbags or straps to hold the electrode in place.
   b. If treating the back, place the electrode under one thigh.

H. Warn the patient that you are going to put some gel (lotion) onto his skin.
I. Apply *room temperature* or cooler coupling medium *liberally* and directly onto the skin:
   1. Protect any remaining clothing from the coupling medium.
   2. *Never* warm up the coupling medium.
   3. Too much coupling medium is better than too little.
   4. Warn the patient, and using the transducer, spread the coupling medium over the skin.
   5. Do *not* place the coupling medium container on top of the unit.
J. Recheck to be sure all intensity controls are off.
K. Turn on the unit (unless preheated).
L. Set the automatic timer to the desired treatment time. Treatment time is usually five minutes.
M. Warn the patient that you are going to turn on the current.
N. With the transducer constantly moving, slowly increase the current intensity until the patient feels a prickly sensation.
O. Move the transducer in small circular or longitudinal strokes over the suspect area. A true trigger point will be quite painful and can be distinguished from the sensation of the current or the muscle contraction.
P. If trigger points are to be treated with ultrasound:
   1. Slowly decrease the current intensity.
   2. Switch to tetanic current if available.

3. Warn the patient.
4. With the transducer moving, slowly increase the current intensity until the patient feels a prickly sensation.
5. Turn on the ultrasound.
6. With the transducer *moving* at a *right angle* to the skin and in light but complete contact, increase the ultrasound intensity to no more than 1 w/cm².

Q. Move the transducer in small circles or longitudinal strokes until the end of the treatment time.

## III. Terminating the Treatment

A. A few seconds before the automatic timer shuts off the unit, with the transducer moving, *slowly* reduce the current intensity to zero and then the ultrasound intensity to off.
B. Wipe off the coupling medium from the transducer and the patient.
C. Turn off the unit.
D. Thoroughly check the patient's skin.

## Chapter 38

# INTERMITTENT COMPRESSION

## *I. Preparations*

A.  Determine the procedure to be used:
1.  The patient's position. Complete relaxation and proper support are absolutely necessary due to the length of the treatment.

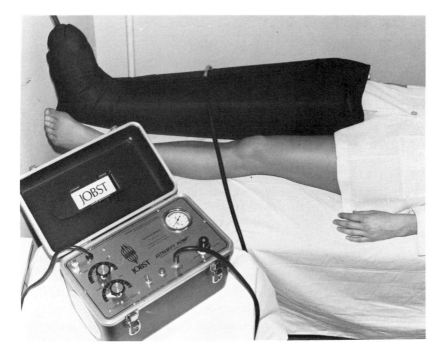

Figure 43. Jobst intermittent compression unit. (Courtesy of Jobst Institute, Inc.)

2.  Pressure readings. These will vary from 30 mm of mercury to 90 mm of mercury.

277

3. Treatment time. Treatment time will vary from two hours to twelve hours.
4. On/off time. The inflation and deflation cycles will be determined by the unit (some units do not have a cycle time switch) or by the condition of the patient.

B. Check the unit:
1. Know how to operate the unit.
2. All dials should be off. Be sure to check the pressure control.
3. Set the recycling timer to the desired pressure and exhaust cycle times.

C. Have all materials ready to use:
1. Pillows will be needed for support and for elevating the extremity.
2. Stockinette or a cotton stocking to go over the extremity for hygienic purposes and to absorb perspiration.
3. Pneumatic appliance.
4. Drape sheet.

## II. Starting the Treatment

A. The patient should evacuate bowels and bladder.
B. Explain the procedure to the patient:
1. Show him the stockinette and tell him what it is for.
2. Show him the pneumatic appliance and how it works.
3. Explain the sensation he *should* feel:
   a. The sensation should be one of pressure.
   b. He may experience some slight discomfort at first, but this should disappear after a few minutes. If it does not, he should tell you.
   c. There should be no pain or tingling in the hand (foot).
   d. There should be no discomfort or pain in the shoulder (hip).
   e. Any discomfort anywhere should be reported to you.
4. Tell the patient how long the treatment will be. Usually the treatment will last for at least two hours. As he

adjusts to the pressure, the treatment time will be extended up to eight to twelve hours.

C. Have the patient remove his clothing:
  1. If he will be sitting, he should remove his shirt (blouse). Do *not* allow him to roll up his sleeve.
  2. If he will be supine, he should remove his trousers, shoes and shirt to prevent his clothing from becoming wrinkled.
  3. Be sure to keep the patient properly draped.
  4. Be sure the patient is warm throughout the treatment.
D. Place the patient in a position that will be comfortable throughout the entire treatment:
  1. If the upper extremity is being treated:
    a. The patient may be sitting or supine. For treatments longer than one hour, the supine position will allow for more relaxation.
    b. The extremity should be flexed higher than the head if possible and abducted slightly to allow for inflation of the appliance.
    c. Use pillows to help support the extremity.
    d. If the patient is sitting, his feet should rest comfortably on the floor. A footstool may be necessary.
  2. If the lower extremity is to be treated:
    a. The patient should be supine.
    b. The hip should be flexed and abducted. Care must be taken to avoid hyperextension of the knee.
    c. Place pillows under the head and opposite knee.
E. Place the extremity in the stockinette:
  1. If treating the upper extremity, the forearm should be supinated in the appliance. Remove all rings, bracelets and watches. If rings cannot be removed, they may be padded with gauze to prevent tearing the stockinette or appliance.
F. Put on the pneumatic appliance:
  1. Be sure the stockinette does not slip.
  2. If you tie the cord on the proximal end of the appliance, be sure it will not be too tight when the appliance is inflated.

G. Connect the appliance to the pressure outlet system on the unit by pushing the tubes together.
H. Turn on the unit. The indication light will glow.
I. Warn the patient that you are about to turn on the pressure.
J. Increase the pressure:
   1. Turn the pressure knob clockwise three or four times.
   2. The unit must be on the inflation cycle before there will be a meter reading.
   3. Wait until you get a reading on the meter *before* increasing the pressure.
   4. Repeat until the desired pressure readings are attained.
K. Remain with the patient through at least three full inflation and deflation cycles to be sure the correct pressure is maintained.
L. Reassure the patient that his circulation will not be cut off, and check for any discomfort.
M. If the treatment is to be long, turn off the unit and remove the appliance every two hours to allow the patient to move around (if indicated) for ten to fifteen minutes.

### III. Terminating the Treatment

A. Turn the pressure down to zero when the unit is on the exhaust cycle.
B. Turn off the unit.
C. Disconnect the appliance from the unit and move the unit out of the patient's way.
D. Remove the appliance and stockinette.
E. Check the skin to see if there were any pressure points caused by wrinkles in the stockinette.
F. The stockinette should be washed before it is used on another patient, or discarded.

## Chapter 39

# COMBINED MOIST HEAT AND ELECTRICAL STIMULATION

## Medcotherm: Medco Products Company, Inc.

### *I. Preparations*

A. Determine the procedure to be used:
   1. Pad application.
   2. Pulsed or tetanizing current.
   3. Cycle rate.
B. Check the unit:
   1. Know how to operate the unit.
   2. Test the unit on yourself.
   3. Unit should be grounded.
   4. All connections should be tight.
   5. All dials should .be off.
   6. Warm up the unit.
C. Have all necessary materials ready to use such as the electrodes, pads, water, gauze, towels, etc.

### *II. Starting the Treatment*

A. Explain the procedure to the patient:
   1. He will feel heat that should be comfortably warm and not hot.
   2. He will feel a mild prickly sensation when the current intensity is increased.
   3. He should tell you immediately if any discomfort occurs.
B. Check the area to be treated:
   1. Skin sensation should be normal. If sensation is not normal, use the lowest current and heat intensities.

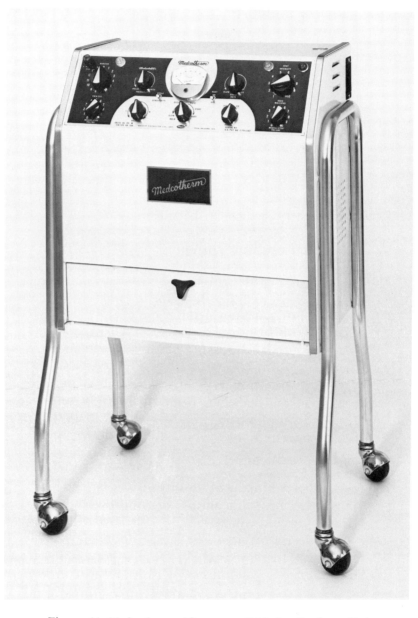

Figure 44. Medcotherm. (Courtesy of Medco Products Co.)

2. The skin should be clean and free from oils, lotions, creams, etc.

3. Avoid treating over abrasions, recent scar tissue or new skin.

C. Never use the electrical stimulations:

1. On any part of any patient who has an external or implanted pacemaker of any kind.

2. Directly over or through the heart.

3. Directly over, through or near a recent or nonunion fracture site.

D. Remove or insulate any metal in the treatment field.

E. Twin Pad/Multipad Application:

1. Soak all sponge pads in warm water.

2. Gently squeeze out the excess water, but leave the pads thoroughly wet.

3. Cover all pads with several layers of wet gauze or toweling for hygienic reasons.

4. Insert the pads in their holders.

5. Protect any clothing and linen from the water.

6. Check to be sure all intensity controls are off.

7. Place the patient on the multipads with the lead cords toward the head and the wide edges toward the outside. This is to assure the proper operation of the left and right sides of the balance control.

8. Place the twin pads as desired.

9. Turn the automatic timer to the desired or prescribed treatment time. Treatment time is usually twenty to thirty minutes.

10. Warn the patient that you are going to turn on the heat.

11. Ask the patient to tell you when he first begins to feel any warmth.

12. Slowly increase the heat intensity until the patient feels the warmth.

13. Set the Medcolator Frequency control to either *pulse* or *tetanize.*

14. Turn Cycle Rate control to *start.*

15. Adjust Cycle Rate control to *slow* or *fast.*

16. Warn the patient you are going to turn on the current.
17. Ask him to tell you when he begins to feel a prickly sensation.
18. *Slowly* increase current intensity to the patient's tolerance: Use the Twin Pad Medcolator Volume control *and* the Quad/Multipad Medcolator Volume controls.
19. The Balance control will concentrate more intensity on either side of the Multipads.
20. When using the Multipads, treatment may be concentrated on only one area:
    a. Turn the Cycle Rate control to *hold* when the desired area is reached.
    b. The numbers 1 through 7 on the meter indicate the pad level where the treatment will be concentrated.
    c. Treatment may also be concentrated in only one area by using the Surge Off/On switch and adjusting the Surge Rate control instead of using the *hold* position on the Cycle Rate control.
F. Twin Pad/Quad Pad Application:
    1. The Twin pads are usually placed on the area of pain and the Quad pads on the back.
    2. Moisten and cover the sponge inserts as previously.
    3. Insert the pads in their holders and place them on the patient.
    4. Warn the patient you are about to turn on the current.
    5. Ask him to tell you when he begins to feel a prickly sensation.
    6. Adjust the current intensity to the patient's tolerance by using the Twin Pad and Quad Pad controls.
    7. Adjust the Pulse Frequency to *tetanize.*
    8. Turn on the Surge On/Off switch.
    9. Adjust Surge Rate control as desired.
    10. The meter will register the intensity and surge frequency when the Cycle Sens switch is in the *sens* position.

### III. Terminating the Treatment

A. A few seconds before the automatic timer goes off, slowly

decrease the current intensity controls to *zero*.
B. Decrease the heat intensity to *zero*.
C. Turn all switches to *off*:
1. If the unit is going to be used again the same day, leave the heat intensity switch on (as indicated by the amber light) to avoid preheating time.
2. The pads must be placed face to face.
D. Remove all pads from the patient.
E. Dry the skin thoroughly.
F. Check the skin.

## *IV. Notes*

A. Remove the sponge inserts each night.
B. These should be washed once a week with soap and warm water.

*Chapter 40*

# MASSAGE

## *I. Preparations*

A. Determine the procedure to be used:
   1. Patient position.
   2. Use techniques that will accomplish the objectives of massage.
B. Have all materials ready to use:
   1. Pillows, rolled towels, etc. for support of the part.
   2. Massage media.
   3. Towels to protect any clothing and to wipe off massage lubricant.

## *II. Starting the Treatment*

A. Your position and body mechanics are *very* important:
   1. Sit down whenever possible such as when massaging the hand, forearm and face.
   2. Don't reach. When massaging an entire back, step or shift your weight toward the head instead of leaning forward.
   3. Use a footstool to stand on if the plinth is too high.
B. Your hands:
   1. Wash your hands before giving a massage.
   2. Nails must be short and clean.
   3. Remove rings.
   4. Remove your watch or push it up your forearm if there is any chance it will touch the patient.
   5. Your hands should be dry and warm.
C. Explain the procedure to the patient:
   1. He should tell you if he feels any pain or other untoward symptoms.
D. Position the patient:

1. The patient *must* be relaxed. In order to relax, he must be comfortable.
2. Proper support of the part being massaged is essential.
3. If possible, elevate the extremity being massaged.
4. Any position that makes use of gravity to stretch the part must not make the patient tense due to the stretching.

E. Drape the patient. See Chapter 1.
F. Check the patient's skin:
   1. The skin should be clean.
   2. Avoid massaging over abrasions, cuts, etc.
   3. Be sure the patient is not sensitive to the massage media.
G. Massage media:
   1. Lubricants such as lotions, creams, oils are used primarily to reduce friction and to soften the skin or scar tissue.
   2. Powders such as talcum make kneading strokes easier. Do *not* use on the face or on patients with respiratory problems.
   3. Use unscented media.
   4. Remove oils, creams, etc. with alcohol if indicated. (Do *not* pour alcohol on the patient.)
   5. Never put the lubricant directly on the patient without warning him first.
H. Massage techniques:
   1. Effleurage — sliding over the skin. Effleurage may be light or heavy pressure:
      a. Used as a preliminary to other massage techniques, sometimes used between other techniques and used to end the treatment.
      b. Hands should be relaxed:
         1. On large areas, use the palms of the hands with the fingers together.
         2. On small areas, use the thumb and fingers.
      c. The movements are long, centripetal strokes.
      d. At the end of the stroke, release all pressure but keep the hands on the skin and return to the starting

       position.
2. Effleurage variations:
   a. Knuckling — deeper than deep effleurage:
      1. Make a fist.
      2. Place the dorsal surface of the first phalanges of the fingers on the part.
      3. Forcefully extend the wrists in a flicking motion.
      4. Proceed in a centripetal direction.
   b. Bilateral tree:
      1. Usually used on the back. Start on the low back and progress toward the head.
      2. Place the hands on the low back with the fingers together, palms next to (not on) the spine and fingers pointing laterally.
      3. The stroking is done laterally and progressing up the spine.
      4. The hands are removed after each stroke.
   c. Shingles — one stroke on top of the previous stroke like shingles on a roof:
      1. Place one hand on the part and move the hand toward you.
      2. As that hand completes the stroke, place the other hand where the first hand started. As one hand finishes the stroke, the other is starting the stroke.
      3. Progress up the part.
   d. Fulling — one hand pushes while the other hand pulls:
      1. Useful on the low back and muscular areas.
      2. Use the palms and fingers.
      3. If used on the low back, face the patient.
      4. Place one hand on the far side of the low back with the fingers pointing laterally.
      5. Place the other hand (with the fingers pointing medially) on the near side of the low back.
      6. The far hand is then pulled toward you as the near hand is pushed away from you.
      7. Do not put pressure on the spinous processes as the hands meet and cross to the opposite side.

3. Petrissage — kneading of the muscles:
   a. Use very little (if any) lubricant.
   b. The hand(s) does *not* slide over the skin, but picks up the muscle and compresses or rolls it against the bone or other muscles.
   c. May be done with one hand or both hands.
   d. The tissues are alternately kneaded between the fingers of one hand and the heel, thenar eminence, and thumb of the other hand.
   e. After four or five movements in one area, progress in a centripetal direction.
4. Petrissage variations:
   a. One hand on small areas such as a child's arm.
   b. One hand on one side of the extremity (biceps) and the other hand on the opposite side (triceps).
   c. The thumb and index finger of one hand.
   d. The thumb of one hand and index finger of the other hand.
5. Friction — skin is moved over the tissues:
   a. Do *not* use lubricants.
   b. Use the tip of a finger or tips of all fingers, ball of the thumb, or heel of the hand.
   c. The skin is moved in small circles over the underlying tissues.
   d. The greatest pressure is applied over the lower part of the circle circumference.
   e. Do three or four circles in one spot and progress upward.
   f. Friction may be done across or along the muscle fibers.
   g. Increase pressure in accordance with patient's tolerance. (Use one finger [hand] on top of the other finger [hand]).
6. Tapotement — percussion of the tissues:
   a. Raindrops — light percussion done with the fingertips as if using a typewriter.
   b. Tapping — done with the volar surface of the fingers (fingers extended), alternating hands in rapid

succession.

c. Slapping — use the palm and fingers, alternating hands in rapid succession.

d. Cupping — same as slapping only the hands are cupped.

e. Hacking — with the palms facing each other and fingers relaxed, use the ulnar borders of the hands in rapid succession.

f. Beating — same as hacking except the fingers are flexed (fist).

g. Pincemont — rapid and gentle pinching of the tissues between the thumb and index finger.

7. Vibration — the hand is placed on the skin and a tremulous movement is applied.

I. Treatment time will vary according to the area treated, objectives to be attained, age and condition of the patient, etc.

## III. Terminating the Treatment

A. End the treatment with light effleurage.
B. Remove the lubricant (if indicated).
C. Give the patient his clothes and tell him to dress.

# SELECTED EQUIPMENT MANUFACTURERS

## I. COLD PACKS

A. Chattanooga Pharmacal Co., P.O. Box 4265, Chattanooga, Tennessee 37405.
B. Cramer Products, Inc., P.O. Box 1001, Gardner, Kansas 66030.
C. Cryomed Devices, Inc., 14 Farber Rd., Princeton, New Jersey 08540.
D. Jack Frost Labs., 3210 Industrial 33rd St., Fort Pierce, Florida 33450.
E. Kwik Kold, 808 Highway 24 West, Moberly, Missouri 65270.
F. Logan, Inc., 16952 Milliken Av., Irvine, California 92705.
G. Nortech Laboratories, 2468 N. Jerusalem Rd., North Bellmore, New York 11738.
H. Physicians and Nurses Manufacturing Corp., P.O. Box 68, Larchmont, New York. 10538

## II. ELECTRICAL STIMULATION AND TESTING UNITS

A. Birtcher Corp., 4501 North Arden Drive, El Monte, California 91731.
B. Burdick Corp., Milton, Wisconsin 53563.
C. Dynawave Corp., 804 W. Main, Batavia, Illinois 60510.
D. Electro-Med Health Industries, Inc., 4506 N. W. 2nd Ave., Miami, Florida 33127.
E. Elmed, Inc., 60 W. Fay Ave., Addison, Illinois 60101.
F. Medco Products Co., Inc., P.O. Box 50070, Tulsa, Oklahoma 74150.
G. Mettler Electronics Corp., 1333 S. Claudina St., Anaheim, California 92805.

H.  Teca Corp., 220 Ferris Ave., White Plains, New York 10603.

## III. HOT PACKS

A.  Chattanooga Pharmacal Co., P.O. Box 4287, Chattanooga, Tennessee 37405.
B.  General Kinetronics Corp., 1270 Broadway, Suite 818, New York, New York 10001.
C.  Jack Frost Labs., 3210 Industrial 33rd St., Ft. Pierce, Florida 33450.
D.  Kwick Kold, 303 Highway 24 West, Moberly, Missouri 65270.
E.  Logan, Inc., 16952 Milliken Ave., Irvine, California 92705.
F.  Nortech Labs., Inc., 2468 N. Jerusalem Rd., North Bellmore, New York 11710.
G.  Physicians and Nurses Manufacturing Corp., P.O. Box 68, Larchmont, New York 10538.

## IV. INFRARED LAMPS

A.  The Burdick Corp., Milton, Wisconsin 53563.
B.  Hydor Therme Corp., 7153 Airport Highway, Pennsauken, New Jersey 08109.

## V. MICROWAVE UNITS

A.  The Burdick Corp., Milton, Wisconsin 53563.
B.  Elmed, Inc., 60 W. Fay Ave., Addison, Illinois 60101.

## VI. SHORT WAVE DIATHERMY UNITS

A.  Birtcher Corp., 4501 North Arden Drive, El Monte, California 91731.
B.  The Burdick Corp., Milton, Wisconsin 53563.
C.  Elmed, Inc., 60 W. Fay Ave., Addison, Illinois 60101.
D.  International Medical Electronics, 2805 Main, Kansas City, Missouri 64108.
E.  Mettler Electronics Corp., 1333 S. Claudina St., Anaheim,

California 92805.

## VII. TANKS

A. Borg-Warner Hospital Therapy Products, Wolf and Algonquin, Des Plaines, Illinois 60018.
B. Market Forge, Everett, Massachusetts 02149.
C. Venutre, P.O. Box 1413, Patterson, New Jersey 07509.

## VIII. ULTRASOUND UNITS

A. Amrex Electronics, 4633 Crenshaw Blvd., Los Angeles, California 90063.
B. Birtcher Corp., 4501 North Arden Drive, El Monte, California 91731.
C. The Burdick Corp., Milton, Wisconsin 53563.
D. Elmed, Inc., 60 W. Fay Avenue, Addison, Illinois 60101.
E. Medco Products Co., Inc., P.O. Box 50070, Tulsa, Oklahoma 74150.
F. Mettler Electronics Corp., 1333 S. Claudina St., Anaheim, California 92805.

## IX. ULTRASOUND GEL

A. Parker Labs., Inc., 103 Elm St., Newark, New Jersey 07105.
B. Pharmaceutical Innovations, Inc., 150 Mt. Pleasant Ave., Newark, New Jersey 07104.

## X. ULTRAVIOLET LAMPS

A. The Burdick Corp., Milton, Wisconsin 53563.
B. Birtcher Corp., 4501 North Arden Drive, El Monte, California 91731.
C. Canrad Precision Industries, Inc., 100 Chestnut St., Newark, New Jersey 07105.
D. Ultraviolet Products, Inc., 5100 Walnut Grove Avenue, San Gabriel, California 91778.

## *XI. WHIRLPOOLS*

A.  Everest & Jennings, 1803 Pontius Ave., Los Angeles, California 90025.
B.  Borg-Warner, Wolf & Algonquin Rds., Des Plaines, Illinois 60018.
C.  Century Manufacturing Co., Industrial Park, Aurora, Nebraska 68818.
D.  Dakon Corporation, 1836 Gilford Ave., New Hyde Park, New York 11040.
E.  Logan, Inc., 16952 Milliken Ave., Irvine, California 92705.
F.  Market Forge, Everett, Massachusetts 02149.
G.  Whitehall Electro Medical Co., P.O. Box 701, Hackensack, New Jersey 07602.

# BIBLIOGRAPHY

## Booklets

1. *Burdick Syllabus*, 7th ed. The Burdick Corporation, Milton, Wisconsin, 1969.
2. *Infrared Therapy*, 2nd ed. The Burdick Corporation, Milton, Wisconsin, 1967.
3. *Microwave Diathermy*, 2nd ed. The Burdick Corporation, Milton, Wisconsin, 1972.
4. *Notes on Low Volt Therapy*. Teca Corporation, White Plains, New York.
5. *Ultrasound*, 4th ed. The Burdick Corporation, Milton, Wisconsin, 1973.
6. *Ultraviolet*, 3rd ed. The Burdick Corporation, Milton, Wisconsin, 1976.

## Books

1. Behrend, Hans J.: Hydrotherapy. In Licht, Sidney H. (Ed.): *Medical Hydrology*. New Haven, Licht, 1966.
2. Finnerty, Gertrude B. and Corbett, Theodore: *Hydrotherapy*. New York, Ungar, 1960.
3. Gucker, Thomas: Heat and cold in orthopedics. In Licht, Sidney H. (Ed.): *Therapeutic Heat and Cold*. New Haven, Licht, 1965, pp. 398-406.
4. Harris, Ronald: Chronaxy. In Licht, Sidney H. (Ed.): *Electrodiagnosis and Electromyography*. New Haven, Licht, 1956, pp. 126-146.
5. Harris, Ronald: Iontophoresis. In Licht, Sidney H. (Ed.): *Therapeutic Electricity and Ultraviolet Radiation*. New Haven, Licht, 1965, pp. 146-168.
6. Karselis, Terrence C.: *Descriptive Medical Electronics and Instrumentation*. Thorofare, Slack, 1973.
7. Knapp, Miland E.: Massage. In Krusen, Frank H. (Ed.): *Handbook of Physical Medicine and Rehabilitation*, 2nd ed. Philadelphia, Saunders, 1971, pp. 381-384.
8. Lehman, Justus F.: Diathermy. In Krusen, Frank H. (Ed.): *Handbook of Physical Medicine and Rehabilitation*, 2nd ed. Philadelphia, Saunders, 1971, pp. 273-345.
9. Licht, Sidney, M.D.: Local cryotherapy. In Licht, Sidney H. (Ed.): *Therapeutic Heat and Cold*. New Haven, Licht, 1965, pp. 538-563.
10. Oester, Y.T. and Licht, Sidney H.: Routine electrodiagnosis. In Licht,

Sidney H. (Ed.): *Electrodiagnosis and Electromyography.* New Haven, Licht, 1956, pp. 109-125.

11. Scott, Bryan O.: Clinical uses of ultraviolet radiation. In Licht, Sidney H. (Ed.): *Therapeutic Electricity and Ultraviolet Radiation.* New Haven, Licht, 1965, pp. 300-343.

12. Scott, Bryan O.: *The Principles and Practice of Diathermy.* Springfield, Thomas, 1957.

13. Scott, Pauline M.: *Clayton's Electrotherapy and Actinotherapy,* 7th ed. Baltimore, Williams and Wilkins, 1975.

14. Shriber, William J.: *A Manual of Electrotherapy,* 4th ed. Philadelphia, Lea & Febiger, 1975.

15. Stillwell, G. Keith: Clinical electrical stimulation. In Licht, Sidney H. (Ed.): *Therapeutic Electricity and Ultraviolet Radiation.* New Haven, Licht, 1965, pp. 104-145.

16. Stillwell, G. Keith: Electrical stimulation and iontophoresis. In Krusen, Frank H. (Ed.): *Handbook of Physical Medicine and Rehabilitation,* 2nd ed. Philadelphia, Saunders, 1971, pp. 374-380.

17. Stillwell, G. Keith: Therapeutic heat and cold. In Krusen, Frank H. (Ed.): *Handbook of Physical Medicine and Rehabilitation,* 2nd ed. Philadelphia, Saunders, 1971, pp. 259-272.

18. Stillwell, G. Keith: Ultraviolet therapy. In Krusen, Frank H. (Ed.): *Handbook of Physical Medicine and Rehabiliation,* 2nd ed. Philadelphia, Saunders, 1971, pp. 363-373.

19. Summer, W. and Patrick, Margaret K.: *Ultrasonic Therapy.* London, Elsevier, 1964.

20. Tappan, Frances M.: *Massage Techniques.* New York, MacMillan, 1961.

21. Thom, Harold: *Introduction to Short Wave and Microwave Diathermy,* 3rd ed. Springfield, Thomas, 1966.

22. Wood, Elizabeth C.: *Beard's Massage — Principles and Techniques,* 2nd ed. Philadelphia, Saunders, 1974.

23. Wynn-Parry, C.B.: Strength-duration curves. In Licht, Sidney H. (Ed.): *Electrodiagnosis and Electromyography.* New Haven, Licht, 1956, pp. 147-176.

24. Zislis, Jack M.: Hydrotherapy. In Krusen, Frank H. (Ed.): *Handbook of Physical Medicine and Rehabilitation,* 2nd ed. Philadelphia, Saunders, 1971, pp. 346-363.

# INDEX

297

with general lamp, 208-214
with local lamps, 197-208
  cold quartz, 197-202
  hot quartz, 202-208
with coal tar, 225-228
Underwater technique with ultrasound, 82-87
and electrical stimulation, 266-272
Unipolar technique, 152-159
Unit, checking of, general considerations for, 10-11
Unwrapped pack, technique of using, 42

**V**

Valuables, patient, 13-14
Vapor coolant sprays, techniques of using, 131-133
Vibration, technique of, 290

**W**

Whirlpools
cold, techniques of using, 115-119
  clothing, removal of, 117
  disinfectant and, 115-116
  patient position, 118
  room temperature for, 115
  turbine and, 116, 118
  water temperature for, 115, 118
warm, techniques of using, 31-37
  cephalic cold and, 32
  clothing, removal of, 33
  cross-infection and, 35
  disinfectant for, 32
  patient position for, 34
  room temperature for, 31
  sterilization of, 37
  swab procedure for, 35-37
  turbine and, 32, 34
  water temperature for, 32